PRAISE FOR *PROTEST KITCHEN*

"*Protest Kitchen* exposes the systemic abuses that result from standard industrialized eating patterns and provides actionable advice for those who empathize with the exploited. This powerful book illustrates how we can resist oppression and create a more just and compassionate world through conscientious food choices."

—Gene Baur, president and cofounder of Farm Sanctuary,
author of *Living the Farm Sanctuary Life*

"In *Protest Kitchen*, Carol J. Adams and Virginia Messina make it very clear how what happens in kitchens, backyards, and other places where food is prepared and consumed has enormous impacts that go way beyond the walls of slaughterhouses, restaurants, and homes. Choosing a plant-based diet is, indeed, a significant form of protest and resistance against a violent, destructive, and discriminatory status quo, and the authors clearly show how personal choices can empower all individuals and make enormous differences not only for the animals and people involved but also for society as a whole."

—Marc Bekoff, author of *The Animals' Agenda: Freedom, Compassion, and Coexistence in the Human Age*
and *Canine Confidential: Why Dogs Do What They Do*

"*Protest Kitchen*'s authors draw on their deep expertise in clinical nutrition and social justice to provide a deeply insightful look at how our food choices can unintentionally support racism, sexism, environmental damage, and other social injustices. Dozens of delicious recipes make it easy to try meals with a lower injustice footprint—my favorites are the imPeach Crumble and the Trumped-Up Cutlets. This wonderful, game-changing book is a must-read for anyone interested in eating mindfully and avoiding collateral damage to society's disenfranchised and marginalized."

—David Robinson Simon, author of *Meatonomics*

"The personal is political—and delicious! *Protest Kitchen* shows you how to change the world . . . one kitchen at a time. When eating is a form of protest, every meal becomes an act of resistance, an opportunity for healing, hope—and Collard Greens with Black-Eyed Peas! Adams and Messina make it fun to align your kitchen with your politics. Go vegan for a day, then a week, then a lifetime."

—Jayne Loader, filmmaker, *The Atomic Café*

"*Protest Kitchen* is a welcome challenge to the world's most ignored social justice space—our own kitchens. Adams and Messina arm hungry advocates with the knowledge needed to bring trips to the grocery store into line with their values, all while providing practical, mouth-watering cuisine to fuel bodies and souls. This delicious page-turner exists in a category of its own. Do yourself a favor and invite *Protest Kitchen* into yours!"

—Chris Sosa, senior editor, AlterNet

"*Protest Kitchen* unpacks the sordid truths associated with our current food system. With action steps and easy and delicious recipes, this book is much more than a cookbook. It will open your mind to how all forms of activism are connected to restructuring food culture."

—David Carter, food justice activist, former NFL player

"*Protest Kitchen* comes at a time when most vegan cookbooks choose to be apolitical—choose not to ask their audience how either collusion with, or resistance against, an oppressive system goes beyond mere taste and desires and begins in the kitchen. Connecting powerful narratives with creative recipes, this book is a much-needed gem for those ready to protest [and cook] against injustices such as speciesism, environmental racism, and misogyny. The personal [palate] is political!"

–Dr. A. Breeze Harper, editor of *Sistah Vegan*

PROTEST KITCHEN

PROTEST KITCHEN

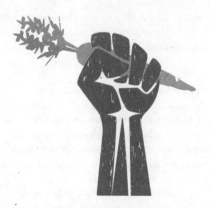

Fight Injustice, Save the Planet, and Fuel Your Resistance One Meal at a Time

CAROL J. ADAMS AND VIRGINIA MESSINA

Conari Press

This edition first published in 2018 by Conari Press, an imprint of
Red Wheel/Weiser, LLC
With offices at:
65 Parker Street, Suite 7
Newburyport, MA 01950
www.redwheelweiser.com

ISBN: 978-1-57324-743-6
Library of Congress Cataloging-in-Publication Data

Names: Adams, Carol J., author. | Messina, Virginia, author.
Title: Protest kitchen : fight injustice, save the planet, and fuel your
resistance one meal at a time / Carol J. Adams and Virginia Messina.
Description: Newburyport, MA : Conari Press, 2018. | Includes bibliographical
references and index.
Identifiers: LCCN 2018018465 | ISBN 9781573247436 (hardback)
Subjects: LCSH: Vegan cooking. | Food preferences--Environmental aspects. |
Sustainable living. | Environmental protection--Citizen participation. |
Green products. | BISAC: SOCIAL SCIENCE / Agriculture & Food. | HEALTH &
FITNESS / Diets. | LCGFT: Cookbooks.
Classification: LCC TX837 .A2925 2018 | DDC 641.5/636--dc23
LC record available at https://lccn.loc.gov/2018018465

Book design by Kathryn Sky-Peck

Printed in Canada
FR

10 9 8 7 6 5 4 3 2 1

IN MEMORY OF OUR MOTHERS

Muriel Kathryn Stang Adams (1914–2009)
and Willie Schrenk Kisch (1923–2002)

and to all who have nurtured children of the resistance

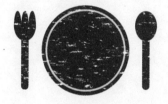

CONTENTS

CHAPTER 3: FOOD JUSTICE 51

CHAPTER 4: TAKE OUT MISOGYNY 69

CHAPTER 5: DREAMING OF AN INCLUSIVE DEMOCRACY 93

CHAPTER 6: CULTIVATING COMPASSION 113

CHAPTER 7: THE DIET YOU NEED NOW 137

CHAPTER 8: FEEDING YOUR RESISTANCE   157

BONUS DAILY ACTION: HOST A COMMUNAL RESISTANCE DINNER   173

THE REPUBLIC IS A DREAM.

NOTHING HAPPENS UNLESS FIRST A DREAM.

Carl Sandburg, "Washington Monument by Night"

WHY A PROTEST KITCHEN?

We live in an unsettled time in politics. Many countries have been roiled by the strength of right-wing and hate groups and the regressive political climate that comes with the airing of those beliefs. As we write this book, tension is growing between countries that are protecting social programs and increasing environmental protections and other countries that are dismantling invaluable social programs and eviscerating environmental protections. Our own country, the United States, is in the latter category.

It's easy to feel overwhelmed. Many of us are concerned about basic human rights, social justice, climate change, and the very future of our democracies. We're marching and protesting, writing letters to our representatives, and volunteering for causes close to our heart. How do we continue without feeling crushed by all there is to do? And how do we not lose hope when every day brings a flurry of news about yet another issue of concern?

There is no shortage of books and websites for those seeking ways to be active and to resist. *Protest Kitchen* is the first resource, however, to suggest that how you eat provides a way to make positive change.

Can something as personal and seemingly disconnected from the world at large as what you're having for dinner have an impact on major issues of our day? The answer is yes. Your food choices are far more powerful than you imagine. In this book, we are going to explore the ways in which a vegan diet, a pattern built around plant foods, can be part of your response *against* misogyny, racism, environmental destruction, and climate change and *for* food justice and compassion. We're going to show you how simple changes to your diet can have a real effect on the environment, but also how food choices celebrate diversity, challenge the patriarchy, and encourage a culture of acceptance, integrity, and honesty. They can also help you care for your own well-being. It may seem like a tall order, but we think that you'll agree, by the time you finish this book, that the simple act of incorporating more vegan food into your daily life can empower your resistance.

We're going to talk about your health a little bit, specifically regarding the dietary changes that can counter feelings of stress. But while a vegan diet can provide remarkable health benefits, this is not one of those books that claims veganism is going to extend your life; it might, but it might not.

Instead, we will show you how veganism is an act of resistance as well as a resource for hope and healing. This is resistance that starts in your kitchen, making it the ultimate in local activism. While most people need to step back from activism now and then out of necessity, everyone has to eat. When the rest of life feels overwhelming, every meal provides an opportunity to continue your resistance.

But what happens in the kitchen doesn't stay in the kitchen. Earlier protestors of unjust conditions knew that. Before the Civil War, abolitionists refused to buy sugar from the slave states. By their mere existence, soup kitchens throughout the decades have protested hunger.

Since the 1960s, boycotts of lettuce, strawberries, and other foods have been an essential part of fighting for better labor conditions for the farmworkers who harvest our food. During that same decade, the Black Panthers began a free breakfast program for schoolchildren. It not only fed more than 20,000 children in nineteen cities, but called attention to the connection between childhood hunger and school performance. In the early 1970s, U.S. housewives stopped buying meat because prices had soared; their boycott prompted slaughterhouses to close for days.

Feeding people and boycotting food linked to unethical practices are the hallmarks of historic protest kitchens.

We know veganism is often seen as *antithetical to* rather than *aligned with* social activism, something for celebrities and those who can afford it, something for health-obsessives, something we just don't have time for. Plenty of negative stereotypes contribute to this view of apolitical vegans: the skinny bitch vegan, the "you-only-think-about-the-animals" vegan, the "holier-than-thou" vegan. Like

> **Feeding people and boycotting food linked to unethical practices are the hallmarks of historic protest kitchens.**

other stereotypes, these woefully miss more than they capture about veganism in the 21st century. They overlook the dynamic variety of vegan social justice activists—the organizing vegans supporting farmworkers, the policy wonk vegans pushing to educate about climate change, the reproductive rights vegan activists who work for access to reproductive health care, the food justice vegans organizing community gardens and food collectives to bring vegan food to their low-income communities, the scientists and inventors seeking to create alternative meats to make eating animal flesh obsolete. Specifically, the stereotypes diminish the meaning of veganism and miss the fact that it is a social justice movement with deep connections to political resistance.

In addition, the stereotypes imply that vegans have deviated from conventional food practices in ways that exclude many. But when you consider the diversity of the places from which we derive some of our favorite foods, a diet often viewed as "exclusive" could be seen as truly "inclusive." We are drawing on the rich soy cultures of China (tofu), Indonesia (tempeh), and Japan (miso and soy milk); the legume protein inventions of the Middle East (hummus and falafel); and the nutrient-dense foods from Latin America (quinoa, black beans, chia seeds, peanuts).

We don't claim that being vegan is all you need to do to make things better in our world. But we do want to show how the practice of veganism and its relationship to how we think about the status of animals are connected to progressive values. Like the #GrabYourWallet campaign, veganism is in part a sophisticated boycott using economic consequences to bring about change.

We will examine how animal oppression is related to human oppression and how changing the way we look at animals and removing barriers of otherness fortify our ability to view all beings (including all people) with respect.

WHAT THE RESISTANCE CAN LEARN FROM VEGANS

Vegans are well versed in local and grassroots activism. We are experienced in working against the propaganda that threatens free speech, a free press, and democracy because that same kind of propaganda has been used to promote a diet of meat and dairy.

Vegans know about compassion fatigue and activism overload and have experience in seeking remedies for both. In fact, our diet might even be a remedy itself.

Veganism is a way to enhance our own lives while honoring and improving the planet and the lives of other humans and animals. At its most basic, vegan choices provide daily reminders that we are connected to each other and that, now more than ever, caring about others is a part of what it means to be living as a global citizen. When you choose a plant-based diet, you're doing good in a myriad of ways *at once*. We will be showing you how and why.

THIRTY DAYS OF ACTION

Protest Kitchen is divided into chapters focusing on democratic principles, climate change, sexual politics, food justice, cultivating compassion, and self-care. Each chapter explores one of these topics as it interacts with diet, lifestyle choices, and conceptualizations and treatment of animals. The chapters reveal the ways in which vegan choices act as resistance and/or inform our resistance. We also provide a short primer on plant-based nutrition for those who wish to move toward a more vegan diet.

But it is one thing to know and another to act on what you know. As we explore these issues, we're going to share ways for you to put the information into practice through thirty days of actions. We'll share helpful phone apps, simple food substitutions, and recipes aimed at putting the daily actions into practice. You can move between insights and ingredients, between reading and recipes, just as in real life we eat and we protest. We're just trying to show you that *how you eat is a form of protest*. The daily actions provide practical options for moving toward more

> **Your food choices are far more powerful than you imagine.**

plant-based foods and also serve as acts of resistance radiating out of the kitchen or as acts of self-care and healing. We know that you may not do all of these daily actions or perhaps you will attempt them over a longer period of time than thirty days. That's okay. This is not meant to be a rigid program. Rather, it's a way of exploring food choices that serve as steps toward aligning your kitchen with your politics.

In offering these suggestions, we are not saying that acting as individuals is all we need to do, but acting as individuals in decisions about our daily food choices is not immaterial and is something we *can* all do.

During a time when you may feel disempowered, your food choices can be a source of empowerment. Our lives are a meaningful stand against injustice, and we can make meaningful choices every day.

Veganism offers a daily way to enact your values, while helping to protect the environment and enhance your health. It becomes a daily reminder that change is possible.

Social change is not just something we must work for; it's something that constantly asks us to change. We know change can be hard. *Protest Kitchen* is here to help. Together we can accomplish so much.

chapter 1

HOW WE GOT HERE

NOSTALGIA, KITCHENS, AND REGRESSIVE POLITICS

Shortly before the 2016 U.S. presidential election, polling revealed that two-thirds of Republicans and a slim majority of independents wanted to return to the 1950s. They believed that U.S. society and its way of life had only gotten worse since then. But two-thirds of Democrats said that things had changed for the better since the 1950s.

The word *nostalgia* combines two Greek roots, *nostos* and *algos* that mean "return home" and "pain." But, nostalgia applies to more than travelers who are homesick. Something *now* evokes nostalgia for *then*.

The voters who longed for the 1950s were *against* the social change that had ushered in new freedoms for many disenfranchised people. They were *for* conservative norms for women. Many believed that it was white people who were the oppressed. To them, the 1950s offered a picture of family and political stability, accompanied by economic growth and prosperity.

According to those who idealize the fifties, it was a time when one lived in a home surrounded by friendly neighbors and with a mother who provided stability and great meals. But the mother in this nostalgic vision is white, and she might have preferred to be working in the plant she was forced out of after World War II. Many forms of birth control taken for granted in the 21st century, like the pill, were not available. Perhaps she didn't want those three or four children to whom she is serving hamburgers and glasses of milk at dinnertime. Blacks were prevented from being in the suburbs by friendly neighbors turned violent. Migrant laborers of Mesoamerican descent labored in fields planting and harvesting crops. They had no health insurance and lived in substandard housing provided by the farmers. And the meat and dairy that filled the 1950s kitchen came increasingly from factory farms. Information from the federal government and advertising—and even school promotions—claimed these were the foods essential to health.

But depending on animal foods for protein, calcium, and other nutrients is a relatively modern concept. This meat- and dairy–focused menu reflects an aberration in, not a continuation of, the world's food-ways. It's also a menu that evolved through decades of oppression that brought us to the less-than-ideal 1950s and beyond.

MEAT AND DAIRY IN THE AMERICAS

Before the 19th century the only people consuming any substantial amount of meat were the royalty and aristocracy of Europe. There were no cows on the land we know as North and South America until the Spanish colonists arrived. Dairy foods were unknown among Meso-americans or Native Americans or First Nations individuals. The pre-Conquest Mesoamericans hunted for meat, but their diets also made generous use of plant foods. Staples, depending on the region, were beans, corn, squash, potatoes, wild greens, nopals (prickly pear cactus), fresh fruit, nuts, and seeds.

When they hauled captured Africans across the ocean in what is known as the Middle Passage, European slavers stocked African crops aboard their ship, believing that familiar food would reduce mortality. Among the foods that Africans contributed to the world food sup-plies are millet, sorghum, coffee, watermelon, black-eyed peas, okra, palm oil, the kola nut, tamarind, and hibiscus. While the African crops brought onboard had no material value for the slave ship captains once they arrived in the Americas, Middle Passage survivors managed to do something extraordinary. They protected their foodways.

Stories passed down through the generations tell how African women, pressed into kitchen duty on the slave ships, hid rice in their own and their children's hair and thus helped in the diffusion through-out the Americas of African foods and dietary practices. The foods that provided the cornerstone for West African foodways were plantains, rice, yams, and millet. Cultivating crops, and preparing foods during slavery, Africans and then African Americans created, as historian James McWilliams calls them, "cuisines of survival."

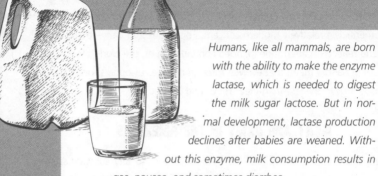

Humans, like all mammals, are born with the ability to make the enzyme lactase, which is needed to digest the milk sugar lactose. But in normal development, lactase production declines after babies are weaned. Without this enzyme, milk consumption results in gas, nausea, and sometimes diarrhea.

Somewhere between 10,000 and 20,000 years ago, a mutation occurred that caused certain northern European populations to become "lactase persistent." They developed a unique ability, by global standards, to digest milk as adults.

The ability to drink large amounts of milk, like the quantities recommended in U.S. food guidelines, is mostly a northern European trait. It wasn't until the 1970s that medical experts recognized that some people had a reduced ability to digest the milk sugar lactose. But to be lactose intolerant is not a deficiency. It's normal. Nearly all Asians and Native Americans and a majority of African Americans, Mexican Americans, and Ashkenazi Jews have low levels of lactase.

The current U.S. Food Guide, called My Plate, continues to provide a culturally narrow perspective by including a dedicated dairy group. Tips for those who can't digest milk and information on plant sources of calcium are relegated to the fine print. This is the influence, at least in part, of a strong dairy lobby in the United States.

Most of the world's population developed food cultures that depend on leafy green vegetables, nuts, seeds, and legumes for calcium. Food guides need to reflect the varied plant-based approaches developed throughout the centuries. National food guides should not be built around recommendations that reflect northern European culture, while expecting that the rest of the population will tweak as needed to meet their own needs.

What these groups didn't bring to the table was beef, and this was viewed as part of their downfall. Nineteenth-century writers attributed the success of the colonizers to their meat diet, rather than their use of advanced technologies of violence, lies and deception, and the introduction of diseases like smallpox to populations lacking inherited resistance to these diseases. For instance, 19th-century medical writer George Beard wrote, "Savages who feed on poor food are poor savages [sic], and intellectually far inferior to the beef-eaters of any race."

Europeans brought cows with them when they came to North America. Jeremy Rifkin, author of *Beyond Beef,* calls cows "hooved locusts" because of the destruction done to the land by these quadrupeds. In order to graze their cows, New England colonists enclosed the land for pasture, supplanting food practices of indigenous people. In the Midwest, open prairie land where buffaloes had roamed became pasture. Traditional patterns of indigenous people prized plant foods and used small amounts of meat for fat and flavor, but they were pushed aside in favor of a meat-centric diet. But it wasn't until the middle of the 20th century that these efforts accelerated to produce the factory farming that is the norm in many countries, including the United States and Great Britain (and increasingly so in China).

FACTORY FARMS

During World Wars I and II in many Western countries, abstaining from meat consumption was a patriotic duty, albeit a mandated one. Meat was rationed and restaurants were required to observe meatless days. In the United States, the burger chain White Castle investigated meatless hamburgers, including a soy burger in the 1940s (an enterprise they revisited more than seventy years later when vegan sliders appeared on their menu in 2015). Newspapers offered recipes for soy burgers and bean burgers.

The end of the war brought prosperity and plenty, which for citizens of the United States meant putting meat and eggs back on the menus in kitchens and restaurants. In the 1950s, the hamburger franchise took off. The "drive-in" with its meat and dairy-centered meals became iconic.

Fueling the demand for meat was a new industrial model for raising animals who become food. It reduced the amount of land needed to grow animals and eventually required less labor as automated systems were introduced. Animals were brought in from the pasture and crowded together in warehouse-like buildings.

Chickens were the first animals to enter the factory farm. At first laying hens, those bred to produce eggs, were housed one per cage. Then they were crowded together within a cage, and then the cages were stacked one on top of another. Now the largest producers grow tens of thousands in one place.

As farms turned into factories, animals were turned into machines. A 1976 article in *Hog Management* magazine advised, "Forget the pig is an animal. Treat him just like a machine in a factory." The manager of Wall's Meat Company defended the use of steel-barred cells called "farrowing crates," which enclose nursing sows in a space so small that they can't turn around. He said, "The breeding sow should be thought of as, and treated as, a valuable piece of machinery, whose function is to pump out baby pigs like a sausage machine."

Chickens, too, are stripped of any moral concern and turned into machines. "The modern layer is, after all, only a very efficient converting machine, changing the raw material—feedstuffs—into the finished product—the egg, less, of course, maintenance requirements," was the observation of one farm magazine.

Before factory farming, cows at least got a break from milking while they were pregnant. But, with a focus on production, expectations for cows changed. Now for seven months each year, they are both pregnant and lactating. They are forcibly impregnated every year because cows don't produce milk unless they have been pregnant. On dairy farms, cows' milk is for profit, not for baby calves. Newborn calves are removed from their mothers soon after birth.

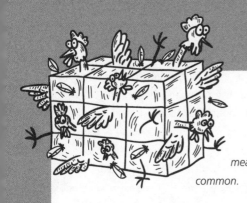

Whether farms are devoted to raising pigs, dairy cows, chickens for eggs, or chickens for meat, certain practices are common.

- **Animals are crowded** into crates or large barns or warehouses, often with barely enough room to turn around.

- **Animals are deprived of the outdoors.** Chickens can't engage in any of their natural behaviors. They can't stretch their wings or dust-bathe or build or sit on a nest. They cannot cluck to their embryos. Even "cage-free" chickens are more often than not housed with little or no access to the outdoors. Most pigs never see the sun or breathe fresh air until they are headed to the slaughterhouse.

- **Animals are denied feed.** Chickens may be starved for up to two weeks to increase egg production. Food is often withheld for as long as twenty-four hours before animals are taken to slaughter. "Skip-feeding" may occur with pregnant or nursing pigs; this involves feeding them every other day.

- **Animals live with unnatural lighting.** Lighting may be kept low to counter the effects of crowding that prompt aggression. In contrast, on egg farms, chickens may be exposed continuously to seventeen hours of light per day to stimulate production.

- **Animals may live in their own waste.** Chickens and pigs must live in their own waste. Ammonia fumes can sting their eyes, burn their lungs, and cause respiratory disease.

While this is all business as usual for the farmers, it's not quite so easy on the cows. Cows miss their calves and they cry and bellow for them. In one town, their calls for their calves so disturbed the residents that many called the sheriff to report "strange noises." The sheriff assured them this was normal for the dairy farm from which the sounds came, but also identified these sounds as cows "lamenting" the loss of their calves. "It happens every year at the same time," one police officer reported.

REGRESSIVE POLITICS

The end of the 1950s saw animals crowded onto factory farms. It also featured racial segregation in cities and suburbs and assumptions about the "family" and a woman's place being in the kitchen (even though many women were working as servants in someone else's kitchen). During World War II, federal policies and day care programs had supported women entering the workforce to replace the men fighting the war. After the war, coercive policies, including the closing of day care programs, sent women workers home. All those Rosie the Riveters were purged from auto plants after World War II. Meanwhile women's rights to function as independent individuals were severely limited: women could not serve on juries in many states, convey property, make contracts, take out credit cards in their own name, or establish residence. African American women were involuntarily sterilized.

As farms turned into factories, animals were turned into machines.

The promise of home ownership in the 1950s was really only fulfilled for white upper-middle-class, and, increasingly in that decade, working-class men. Racially explicit laws, regulations, and government practices created a nationwide system of urban ghettos, surrounded by white suburbs. African Americans seeking to integrate predominantly white neighborhoods were met with phone threats, rocks thrown through their windows, and cross burnings. Through laws reinforced by white violence in the South, African Americans experienced the force of segregation. Rigid Jim Crow laws segregated public spaces and created nearly insurmountable barriers to voting while civil rights activists were killed and their murders went unavenged. In the North, redlining (failure to provide mortgages for people of color wanting to buy houses in white neighborhoods) and restrictive covenants prevented African Americans from joining whites in the suburbs.

The Cold War, the "Red Scare," and McCarthyism created anxiety and justified attacks on and suppressions of speech. Gays and lesbians were persecuted, fired from federal and state jobs because they were viewed as more of a "security risk" than Communists and vulnerable to blackmail by Russians. Women died from self-inflicted and illegal abortions. By the end of the 1950s, a third of U.S. children were poor and medical insurance for older people was absent.

It is true that job security, especially for white men, was greater in the 1950s. Real wages rose, not only for the top earners but also for the bottom 70 percent. At the same time, however, various forms of coercion deprived many women of the opportunity to work. Stephanie Coontz points out in *The Way We Never Were: American Families and the Nostalgia Trap*, "When commentators lament the collapse of traditional family commitments and values, they almost invariably mean the uniquely female duties associated with the doctrine of separate spheres for men and women."

The fifties don't resemble the just society we are working for, and in fact the comforting notion of "the fifties" doesn't resemble the fifties, either. If you lived through the 1950s (or are familiar with more accurate accounts than those provided by TV sitcoms), you know that underneath the veneer of stability and happiness lies the sordid truth of what U.S. democracy was like in that decade. As Coontz wryly puts it, *Leave It to Beaver* was not a documentary.

ANIMAL ACTIVISM AND
21ST-CENTURY REGRESSIVE POLITICS

When we think about regressive politics in the 21st century, three common practices impede positive social change:

1. relabeling information and renaming activism
2. repressing speech
3. targeting activists as terrorists and thereby suppressing activism

It may not seem very obvious to turn our attention to meat and dairy when we are concerned about regressive politics, but believe us when we say vegans have been there and experienced this. Over the past thirty years in working to expose the cruelty of the factory farm, the slaughterhouse, the laboratories that experiment on animals, fur farms, and other businesses, we have been countered by all three of these measures. For example, as animal activists expose the cruelty of factory farms, farmers revise language to describe those practices. Slaughterhouses are "processing plants." Chickens that are crammed into warehouses are "free-range." Pigs confined in gestation crates are kept there for their own "safety."

The success of animal rights activism, accompanied by more radical acts of going undercover in factory farms and sometimes liberating animals, brought this activism to the attention of the federal authorities, especially because they were affecting the bottom line of huge industries. From the corporate viewpoint, something was needed to impede activism's success. The response was passage of Ag Gag laws, some of the earliest repressive legislation of our time.

"Ag-Gag" laws are designed to repress speech. These laws have moved beyond preventing property damage by animal activists to quashing the recording of what is happening on industrial farms and in slaughterhouses. More recent laws simply make it illegal to record animals on farms, even from a distance.

Congress passed the Animal Enterprise Terrorism Act (AETA) in 2006. It was drafted by the conservative and corporate-influenced American

Legislative Exchange Council to expand "the definition of terrorism to include not only property destruction, but any action intended to 'deter' animal enterprises." These included civil disobedience and documenting corporate misconduct. Those involved in drafting the bill included the National Association for Biomedical Research, Fur Commission USA, GlaxoSmithKline, Pfizer, Wyeth, United Egg Producers, and National Cattlemen's Beef Association.

Congressman Dennis Kucinich spoke against the bill, pointing out that existing federal laws were adequate and that "the bill created a special class of crimes for a specific type of protest, and such a broad terrorist label would chill free speech." Traditional acts of nonviolent civil disobedience, among other activities, were now labeled "terrorist."

As author Will Potter points out in his groundbreaking book *Green is the New Red,* some definitions of terrorism have added property violence. (Animals are also viewed as "property.") But if property violence is terrorism, the British suffragettes of the 1910s who destroyed shop windows in London were terrorists. African Americans who freed themselves from bondage were terrorists, sabotaging the slave industry by removing their bodies from it.

The questions of who are terrorists and what terrorism is have gained new relevance as we hit the streets to challenge inhumane policies. Potter warns that "the strategies and tactics used against animal activists aren't going to stop there. They are expanding to Black Lives Matter, to people protesting the Trump Inauguration, the Dakota Pipeline protestors. They are expanding this framing of who is subversive and who is dangerous, and as well, there is an attempt to narrow that discussion in terms of people in power. So that by definition whatever you are doing as a person in power is not part of the debate."

NO TIME FOR NOSTALGIA IN PROTEST KITCHENS

The "traditional" family of the 1950s was a new phenomenon, and the decade was a departure from earlier ones rather than a culmination of trends. For example, in the 19th century, a commitment to domesticity took middle-class women outside the house, improving social conditions for impoverished families. In the 1950s this emphasis on domesticity restricted middle-class women to their home. The amount of time women spent doing housework actually *increased* during the 1950s. People married at a younger age and women bore children earlier and closer together.

Turn-of-the-20th-century feminists challenged the idea of a private kitchen with proposals for communal kitchens, food deliveries, and cafeterias. They recognized the need to reduce the domestic labors of women, especially for those who worked outside the home. Private kitchens were viewed as inefficient ways of preparing food. These proposals for communal food preparation that would relieve individual women of these tasks were forgotten by the 1950s. Husbands typically did any cooking that took place out-of-doors. A man's domain in the suburbs was the backyard barbecue where he grilled meat for a Saturday cookout. Cookbooks maintained this hierarchy of food preparation, reinforcing the idea that men want meat and are the ones who should oversee its cooking on the grill, while women could be happy at a luncheon of salads and preparing food inside.

> **It is time to envision a transformed kitchen— one that serves as a setting for protest, resistance, and nourishment.**

The kitchen, already domesticated, became thoroughly privatized, feminized—and depoliticized. How could protest come from *that* kitchen? We're going to see that it's not only a logical place, but an essential one for protest against regressive politics.

Here's the irony: the fifties are no longer with us in ways that improve our democracy, but the fifties are still with us in ways that we don't realize. We continue to rely on diets built on meat, eggs, and dairy foods. This focus on animals as food is responsible for a host of problems, as we'll see in the chapters ahead. But there is something we

can all do. We can leave nostalgia behind. It is time to envision a trans-
formed kitchen—one that serves as a setting for protest, resistance, and
nourishment.

Daily Action 1:

TASTE TEST NONDAIRY MILK

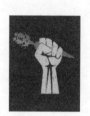

Swapping out cow's milk for milk made from plants is just about the
easiest dietary change you can make. Plant milks are made from soybeans, almonds, coconut, pea protein, rice, hazelnuts, hempseeds, walnuts—even pistachios. You are pretty much guaranteed to find at least
one that you'll like.

Nutrition varies considerably among the different types. For example, both soy milk and milk made from pea protein provide about the
same amount of protein that you'd get from a glass of cow's milk.
In contrast, milks made from nuts (including coconut) and grains are
typically low in protein, although a few brands of almond milk now·
have higher amounts. Milk made from hempseeds or flaxseeds provide
essential fats. Most types of milk are fortified with calcium and vitamin
D at levels that are equivalent to cow's milk. If milk plays a significant
role in your diet, it's a good idea to choose fortified brands. If you are
using milk just in cooking, this doesn't matter as much.

When it comes to drinking a glass of refreshing cold milk, or pouring it over your morning cereal, the only thing that really matters is
which milk tastes best to you and how its nutritional profile fits your
needs. For other uses, certain milks are better choices than others.
The good news is that you can find a plant milk for every possible use
you can think of.

Soy Milk is good for baking because of its higher protein content. It
also works well in sauces, vegan pumpkin pie, puddings, and mashed
potatoes. You can also make buttermilk from soy milk by adding 2
teaspoons of cider vinegar to one cup of soy milk. Let it stand until

it separates. "Light" soy milk is lower in fat and calories and usually sweeter, so it's not always interchangeable with regular full-fat soy milk.

Pea Protein Milk is generally equivalent to soy milk and cow's milk in protein content. Although it has a somewhat thinner consistency, it can generally do anything that soy milk can do.

Almond Milk is probably the most popular vegan milk on the market. Because of its slightly sweet flavor, it's a favorite for smoothies and is a good choice for desserts. Depending on the brand (and your taste), it may be too sweet for savory sauces.

Coconut Milk is somewhat higher in fat than most other plant milks. Although this kind of milk works well in baked goods, it may not be the best choice for puddings and custards since the fat may separate and create a greasy texture. Coconut milk beverages also have a slight coconut flavor, so you'll need to consider that if you want to use it in recipes. Note that the coconut milk sold as a beverage in the dairy case is different from the culinary coconut milk in a can. Canned coconut milk—even the "lite" version—is extremely high in fat and very thick and creamy. It's wonderful for making curried dishes or to use in desserts, but you wouldn't want to drink it.

Rice Milk has a thin consistency and is usually sweet. If you choose to use it on your morning oatmeal, you'll probably find that you can skip adding any other sweeteners. It's generally not a good candidate for baked goods or for savory sauces.

Hempseed Milk has a creamy texture and a rather distinctive flavor, making it better suited to savory dishes than desserts.

Flax Milk has a somewhat thin, smooth consistency. It's a good addition to smoothies or to make creamy desserts. Unsweetened flax milk can also be used in savory sauces.

COOKING WITH PLANT MILKS

Baked Goods	Puddings and Custards	Mashed Potatoes	Savory Sauces
• Soy • Pea • Coconut • Oat	• Soy • Pea • Cashew	• Soy • Pea • Cashew	• Soy • Pea • Coconut • Hemp • Oat • Cashew

Smoothies	In Coffee	To Make Buttermilk	For Drinking
• Soy • Pea • Almond • Coconut • Cashew • Rice	• Soy • Cashew	• Soy	• Any milk you enjoy

GOOD NUTRITION FROM PLANT MILKS

Protein (similar amounts to cow's milk)	Moderate Levels of Protein	Omega-3 Fats	Calcium and Vitamin D
• Soy • Pea	• Some brands of almond milk • Oat • Hemp	• Hemp • Flax	• Any milk that is fortified with these nutrients (most are)

Oat Milk has a mild flavor and the consistency of low-fat cow's milk. It's somewhat higher in protein than nut milks and a good choice for savory sauces and baking.

Cashew Milk is somewhat less sweet than almond milk (which is only very slightly sweet anyway) and can be a good choice for savory dishes like vegan fettuccine Alfredo.

• • •

Use our chart on page 21 as a general guide for how to use different plant milks, but keep in mind that these are suggestions rather than rules. Experiment with the plant milks you enjoy in your favorite recipes to find what works for you.

Creamed Spinach

Makes 4 servings

Use mild-flavored baby spinach in this recipe to make it an inviting choice for kids (or anyone who is not a vegetable fan). If you don't have fresh spinach or want an even faster recipe, use frozen chopped spinach. Defrost it and squeeze all of the water out. It doesn't need to be cooked first. Just add it to the sauce and heat until hot.

    10-ounce bag of baby spinach
    1 tablespoon vegan butter or extra-virgin olive oil
    1 medium shallot, diced
    ½ tablespoon all-purpose flour
    ½ cup soy milk
    ¼ teaspoon ground nutmeg
    ½ teaspoon salt
    ⅛ teaspoon freshly ground black pepper

- Add the spinach to pot of boiling water. Simmer 1 minute. Drain and press the water out.

- Melt the butter or heat the olive oil over medium heat. Add the shallot and cook until translucent—about 3 minutes. Add the flour and cook, stirring constantly, for 1 minute.

- Add the soy milk, nutmeg, salt, and pepper, then raise the heat to high and cook, stirring constantly, until thickened.

- Add the spinach, and stir to combine.

Vegan Irish Cream

Makes 24 1½ ounce servings

Bailey's uses almond-based ingredients to create a vegan version of their signature liqueur. But you can save money and achieve an even richer drink in just a few minutes. Using a blend of cashew milk and coconut milk (this is the canned coconut milk used in cooking, not the type you drink) gives it creaminess without coconut flavor.

½ cup cashew milk
1 cup Irish whiskey
¾ cup granulated sugar
1 can full-fat coconut milk
1½ teaspoons cocoa
¾ teaspoon pure vanilla
¼ teaspoon instant coffee

Combine all the ingredients in a blender and blend on high until smooth and creamy. Let the mixture sit in the refrigerator overnight to allow the flavors to marry. Shake before serving.

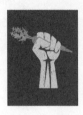

Daily Action 2:

CELEBRATE AMERICAN CUISINE

Vegans love to celebrate foods and recipes from all over the world, and you'll see that we do plenty of that in this book. But let's start with some all-American food using ingredients that are indigenous to the Americas and that have been important in the diet of people here since long before European colonists arrived.

Three Sisters Soup

Makes 6 servings

When Europeans came to North America in the early 1600s, Native Americans had been growing corn, beans, and squash for hundreds of years. According to legend, the vegetable trio were known as the "three sisters" and often planted together. The corn provided a structure for the beans to climb while the squash spread over the ground as a living mulch, helping to retain moisture in the soil. The beans replenished the soil and also provided protein in meals. While not an authentic recipe, this soup brings together ingredients with a rich American heritage.

6 cups vegetable stock

2 cups frozen white or yellow corn (or 1 16-ounce can)

1 14-ounce can of kidney or pinto beans, drained and rinsed (or 1½ cups cooked beans)

1 small onion, coarsely chopped

1 rib celery, coarsely chopped

1 15-ounce can of pumpkin puree (not pumpkin pie filling) or one package of pureed frozen butternut squash

½ teaspoon dried sage

½ teaspoon mild chili powder

- Bring the vegetable stock to a simmer. Add the corn, beans, onions, and celery and simmer for 10 minutes.

- Stir in the pumpkin or squash, plus the dried sage and chili. Simmer over low heat for 20 minutes.

Mexican Rice

Makes 4 servings

This traditional Mexican side dish was created by Richard Tamez for the *veganmexicanfood.com* website which is a part of the Food Empowerment Project, a nonprofit organization that seeks to create a more just and sustainable world by recognizing the power of food choices.

1 tablespoon vegetable oil
¾ cup white rice
1 medium tomato, chopped
½ medium onion, chopped
1 tablespoon garlic powder
½ tablespoon salt
1 14.5-ounce can vegetable broth (or equivalent homemade
    vegetable broth)
1 cup water

- Heat the vegetable oil in saucepan over medium to high heat. Once it's hot, pour in the rice and brown evenly. Stir consistently to keep the rice from burning.

- Combine the chopped tomato, chopped onion, garlic powder, and salt in a blender and blend at medium speed for approximately 2 minutes, or until evenly blended. Pour this mixture over the browned rice and stir it until all the rice is coated.

- Pour the vegetable broth and water over the rice but don't stir it. Bring the liquid to a boil, then reduce the heat to low and cover.

Keep an eye on the rice so it doesn't burn but don't stir it. Once all the liquid is gone, after about 20 minutes, turn off the heat and let the rice stand covered for at least 10 minutes before serving.

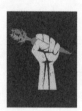

Daily Action 3:

TRY A VEGAN BARBECUE RECIPE

Many vegan foods are at home in a barbecue sauce, but nothing is more fun than making barbecued pulled "pork" from jackfruit. The large fruit of a tropical tree, jackfruit is native to India and widely popular throughout the tropical regions of the world. The unique thing about jackfruit is that you can shred it with your fingers to create a texture that is remarkably like pulled pork. Because its flavor is so mild, it's also a perfect fit for barbecued dishes.

Look for unripe or green jackfruit that is canned in water if possible or in brine. Avoid jackfruit canned in syrup, which will make your pulled "pork" sandwich too sweet.

Pulled "Pork" Jackfruit Barbecue

A quick, tasty way to enjoy a barbecue!

Makes 6 sandwiches

2 20-ounce cans young green jackfruit packed in water or brine
3 tablespoons extra-virgin olive oil
1 cup chopped onion
2 jalapeños or other hot pepper, seeded and minced
2 cups of your favorite barbecue sauce with 2 cups
    water whisked in
Buns for serving

- Rinse the jackfruit, drain, and squeeze out the excess water with your hands. Remove the "core" part of the fruit and discard. Then pull the jackfruit apart. Leave this in a colander to drain.

- Heat the oil and sauté the onion and jalapeños until the onion is soft.

- Stir in the jackfruit. Add the barbecue sauce and water to the jack-fruit. Bring the mixture to a boil, then reduce the heat to simmer. Let this simmer for 45 minutes to one hour, checking to make sure that the sauce does not boil away. The barbecue sauce should be thick.

- Serve on a bun that is grilled or pan-toasted with a little olive oil.

Carrot Dogs

Serves 8—or 4 if you are hungry!

We're not going to pretend that these are exactly like hot dogs, but they are a fun and delicious addition to your next barbecue. Kids especially like them, making it an easy way to convince them to eat their veggies. Serve these on a hot dog bun with grilled onions, mustard, and sauer-kraut or whatever you enjoy. Or slice them into vegetarian baked beans.

8 carrots (choose ones that are similar in size for even cooking)
1 vegetable bouillon cube
½ cup hot water
¼ cup soy sauce
¼ cup apple cider vinegar
1 teaspoon garlic powder
½ teaspoon cumin
½ teaspoon onion powder
1½ tablespoons liquid sweetener (like agave or molasses)
½ teaspoon liquid smoke
Dash of nutmeg
2 tablespoons olive oil, divided

- Trim the tops and bottoms from the carrots.

- In a large skillet, bring enough water to cover the carrots to a boil. Add the carrots and simmer for 6 to 10 minutes until they are soft enough to be pierced with a fork. Don't let them get soft enough to break apart. When the carrots are cooked, drain them and plunge them into a bowl of ice water to prevent them from cooking further.

- While the carrots are cooking, dissolve the bouillon cube in the ½ cup of hot water. Stir in the soy sauce, apple cider vinegar, garlic powder, cumin, onion powder, sweetener, liquid smoke, nutmeg, and 1½ tablespoons of the olive oil.

- Place the carrots in a flat airtight container or large ziplock bag and pour the marinade over them. Let them marinate in the refrigerator for at least 8 hours.

- Heat the remaining ½ tablespoon of olive oil in a skillet. Drain the carrots, reserving the marinade. Add the carrots and ½ cup of the marinade to the skillet. Cook over medium heat until the marinade has evaporated and the carrots are well brown. The marinade will create a nicely caramelized coating.

- Serve immediately.

chapter 2

EATING TO COMBAT CLIMATE CHANGE

Between 2008 and 2018, the United States experienced twice as many record daily high temperatures as record lows. When climate scientists analyzed temperatures from weather stations, they concluded that this increase in record highs is due to global warming. Overall, the world has warmed by 0.85°C over the past 130 years. NASA estimates that temperatures could rise by anywhere between 2 and 6°C by the end of the 21st century.

Those numbers may not sound dramatic, but they are. In fact, they could be catastrophic. Global warming of this magnitude drives climate change, which includes changes in precipitation patterns, increased prevalence of droughts and wildfires, and extreme weather patterns such as heat waves and hurricanes. As ice melts, the oceans are rising, which contributes to erosion along coastal regions and severe flooding. These changes will impact human health, water supply, agriculture, societal stability, and the ecosystem.

We need a comprehensive, global approach to combating climate change, but you also have opportunities to make a difference for the earth and its inhabitants right at home in your own kitchen. Your food choices represent a powerful way to impact global warming and climate change.

CLIMATE CHANGE AND BIODIVERSITY

The impacts of climate change on nature and wildlife are already apparent around the globe. As sea temperatures rise, parts of the Great Barrier Reef off the coast of Australia have begun to die. High levels of carbon dioxide in the atmosphere result in acidification of ocean water, which reduces the ability of corals and other sea life that make up reefs to build shells and skeletons from calcium carbonate.

Some 10,000 miles away Arctic sea ice is also disappearing. More than one-third of the total, or about one million square miles of sea ice in the region, has been lost since the 1980s. The Arctic's year-round ice is expected to shrink to a narrow strip off the northern edge of

Canada and Greenland in the next few decades.

This dramatic change is already affecting polar bears, who need an ice shelf for feeding and must live on their fat reserves during ice-free periods. As these ice-free periods get longer due to warmer temperatures, the polar bear population is shrinking. Some animals can migrate as their territory changes, but polar bears have nowhere to go. "Sea ice really is their platform for life," said Kristin Laidre, a researcher at the University of Washington's Polar Science Center. One estimate is that there will be no polar bears in Alaska in seventy-five years. Sea ice is also disappearing in the Antarctic and with it the ice algae and krill that serve as a major food source for fish, seabirds, and marine mammals.

> **Replacing animal foods with plants is the most effective dietary change you can make for the health of the planet.**

The loss of a few species may not result in immediate obvious changes, but over time, there can be a cascade of repercussions that impact food, water, air, and health care. One example is that a significant drop in the shark population off the East Coast has caused a rise in fish populations that have decimated shellfish in the area. Loss of shellfish has a negative impact on water quality and also on the sea grass beds that are an important feeding ground for turtles. Their dense roots also secure the seabed, providing some storm protection to coastal regions.

So far biologists have identified about a million and a half species that share the planet with us, but they say there may be many millions more that have yet to be identified. This means that we still have a limited understanding of how all of these plants, animals, insects, and bacteria around us interact to maintain a balance among the resources we rely on.

CLIMATE CHANGE IS A HUMAN RIGHTS ISSUE

People in the world's poorest countries are most vulnerable to the impacts of climate change, including rising sea levels, natural disasters, food insecurity, and infectious diseases. Changing rainfall patterns can affect water supplies and water safety. More than half of the world's population depends on glacier melt or snowmelt for water. As higher temperatures reduce glacier mass and cause more rain than snow, this resource will dwindle. Water scarcity is one factor that can lead to famine. Another is the effect of climate change on crop yields. One study found that average yields of eight major crops in Africa and South Asia are expected to decrease by 8 percent by the 2050s due to climate change. In coastal regions, rising sea levels can result in flooding which contaminates drinking water and also creates breeding grounds for insects like mosquitoes that transmit malaria and dengue fever. Poor water quality leads to diarrhea, which kills more than a half-million children every year.

A memorandum on the White House website in September 2016 noted that impacts of climate change had the potential to adversely affect military readiness, negatively affect military facilities and training, and increase demands for federal support in the United States as well as for efforts to support international stability and humanitarian assistance needs. (Any mention of those concerns disappeared after the inauguration in January 2017.)

The independent think tank Adelphi, which focuses on climate change, environment, and development, reports that climate change helps create an environment in which terrorists can thrive and more easily pursue their strategies. A case in point is the rise of the Boko Haram around Lake Chad in northern Africa. Lake Chad is now one-twentieth of the size it was thirty-five years ago. Dwindling resources promote local competition for land and water, fueling social tensions, population displacement, and even violent conflict. Groups like Boko Haram know how to exploit this to their advantage as people—especially unemployed youth with limited prospects—become vulnerable to recruitment.

Clearly, the causes of humanitarian crises in sub-Saharan Africa are complex and multifaceted. Although they are not caused by climate change, by contributing to a more fragile environment climate change worsens the situation.

The issue of climate justice is also relevant to the disability community and to older people. They may have greater medical needs, making them more vulnerable during natural disasters. They are likely to require help in evacuating during hurricanes and floods and wildfires.

CLIMATE CHANGE IS A PROBLEM CAUSED BY HUMANS

There is near unanimous agreement that the current warming of the globe is due to the amount of greenhouse gases in the atmosphere. These gases, which include carbon dioxide, chlorofluorocarbons, methane, and nitrous oxide, trap heat, preventing it from escaping into the outer atmosphere. They come mainly from the burning of fossil fuels (coal, oil, and gas) along with the clearing of forests and agricultural practices.

Reducing greenhouse gas emissions is the key to slowing global warming. This means improving our energy efficiency and using energy sources that produce less or no carbon dioxide. Influencing decisions at the national level is a formidable challenge. But as we work to change national politics, there is much we can do at home. It's our protest kitchen solution, one that many have chosen because they realized it offers the single most effective way to shrink one's own carbon footprint.

PROTEIN FACTORIES IN REVERSE

In her 1971 groundbreaking book *Diet for a Small Planet*, Frances Moore Lappé coined the term "protein factory in reverse" to describe modern meat production. She calculated that for every sixteen pounds of grain and soy fed to beef cattle in the United States we get back one pound of meat. In terms of nutrition, we reclaim just 5 percent of the calories and 12 percent of the protein that is fed to the cow according to her calculations. While the numbers are less dramatic for poultry, milk, and eggs, the relationship holds. Feeding protein and calories to farmed animals is an inefficient use of those resources.

It's not hard to see why this happens. Calories and protein fed to animals don't all go toward the production of muscle, which is what humans end up eating. Much of it is used for energy by the animal or to make some part of the body that we don't eat. It's wasteful, which would be bad enough. What makes it worse is the effect on the planet and on global warming when resources are poured into producing grain and soybeans to feed farmed animals. If we simply ate the grains and beans ourselves, we'd need to grow far less of these crops and we'd save both water and energy. Depending on a number of factors, it can take anywhere from four to twenty-six times as much water and six to twenty times as much fossil fuel to produce animal protein compared to an equivalent amount of soy protein.

> **We have the opportunity to consume in a way that lightens the burden of global warming on the rest of the world.**

It's become common knowledge that plant-based diets exploit fewer resources. When researchers compared the environmental impacts of producing foods consumed by vegetarians and nonvegetarians from California, they found that the meat-eaters' diets required nearly three times more water and thirteen times more fertilizer.

In addition to diverting resources from more sustainable forms of food production, meat, dairy, and egg production does direct damage to the environment through chemical runoff that may cause acidification, algal blooms, and dead zones in lakes and coastal areas. Animals bred for food generate 1.4 billion tons of waste per year or more than five tons of waste for every U.S. citizen. Most of this waste is untreated and contains pathogens that could—and at times have—contaminated food and water supplies.

Since *Diet for a Small Planet* was published, we've come to recognize that the environmental damage associated with the intensive farming practices we talked about in chapter 1 goes beyond squandering of natural resources. These farms contribute to global warming through greenhouse gas emissions that include carbon dioxide emissions from fossil fuel use on the farm or in the supply chain, nitrous oxide emissions from fertilizer application, and methane emissions from the animals themselves.

Although large animals like cows cause the greatest harm to the environment, all animal agriculture is damaging, even fish. Marine ecologist Daniel Pauly of the University of British Columbia says, "While the climate crisis gathers front-page attention on a regular basis, people—even those who profess great environmental consciousness—continue to eat fish as if it were a sustainable practice. But eating a tuna roll at a sushi restaurant should be considered no more environmentally benign than driving a Hummer or harpooning a manatee."

Shrimp farming uses even more energy than production of chicken or beef, largely due to the need for water exchange and aeration. Removing small fish from the ocean and turning them into feed for large carnivorous fish is also affecting marine mammals such as dolphins who depend on these small fish for survival. At the same time, overfishing of large carnivorous fish can upset the balance of the ocean ecosystem in ways that increase carbon dioxide production.

All food production contributes to greenhouse gases, but the difference between the impact of plant foods and animal products is pronounced. The food system is responsible for more than a quarter of all greenhouse gas emissions, but 80 percent of these emissions are associated with livestock production.

And while choosing locally produced foods is a good way to support your community, it doesn't do much to reduce your carbon footprint. Most carbon emissions involving food come from production, not transportation.

Sometimes we hear disheartening information about the state of the world and feel powerless to have any positive impact. But the bad news about climate change is balanced by the good news that we truly have the ability to change the future. It's in our hands—our forks, our spoons, our chopsticks: Replacing animal foods with plants is the most effective dietary change you can make for the health of the planet. When scientists computed the greenhouse gas emissions associated with sixty-one different food categories, they found that with just one exception, all of the biggest contributors were meat or dairy products. Researchers from Loma Linda University in California measured average greenhouse gas emissions from vegans and vegetarians and compared them to emissions from people eating varying amounts of meat or eating fish but no other meat. The less animal food a group ate, the lower the greenhouse gas emissions associated with their diet. Emissions associated with meat-eaters were twice as high as those in vegans.

SOY AND THE AMAZON RAINFOREST

The Amazon rainforest, the largest in the world, has been called "the lungs of the planet" because of its ability to remove carbon dioxide from the air and convert it to oxygen. With rising levels of carbon dioxide in the atmosphere, we need the Amazon more than ever. As farmers clear trees and other vegetation to make room to graze cattle and grow soybeans, the forest is getting smaller and its carbon-reducing abilities are shrinking as well.

One common misconception is that we should stop eating foods made from soybeans since their production contributes to rainforest loss. But the tofu and veggie burgers you eat have nothing to do with the Amazon rainforest, other than the fact that they may help preserve it. Most of the soybeans grown in the Amazon are exported to feed animals on factory farms. It's a dual assault on the environment. Factory farming of animals produces greenhouse gases and at the same time clearing land to grow food for those animals reduces the planet's ability to process the gases. Again, when we consider the "protein factory in reverse" scenario, it makes sense that the way to protect the rainforest is to eat soybeans and other plant foods directly instead of eating the animals who eat the beans.

WHAT TO EAT INSTEAD OF MEAT: BEANS AND BURGERS

One simple change—replacing beef with beans—could have a dramatic impact on greenhouse gas emissions. That's the conclusion of researchers from four universities who teamed up to measure the effects. Even if nothing else changed, replacing beef with beans would allow the United States to achieve between 46 and 74 percent of the reductions needed to meet 2020 emission goals. Substituting beans for beef would also free up 42 percent of U.S. cropland currently under cultivation. Although this study looked at the effects of dietary change among the U.S. population, the findings clearly apply to any population where meat plays a central role in diets.

Because they are rich in protein and have a small carbon footprint, meals built around beans represent a remarkable response to global warming. Not only do beans take less from the earth, but by fixing nitrogen in the soil, they give back to the earth what other crops deplete.

Making the switch to more processed types of plant proteins like veggie burgers and other plant-based meats is somewhat less impactful than eating beans. Food processing itself requires energy and contributes to global warming. But even foods that involve some processing, like soy milk, tofu, and veggie burgers, produce far fewer greenhouse gases than comparable animal foods.

COMBATING CLIMATE CHANGE: IT'S UP TO US

Worldwide meat production has increased 20 percent in just the last ten years. People in industrial countries consume the most meat, nearly double the amount as people in developing countries.

Many of us are in the uniquely privileged position of being able to choose what we will eat, something that is certainly not an option for much of the world's population. Because the impacts of our habits are felt around the world and the impacts of climate change affect the world's poorest people who have the fewest resources to respond, this privilege presents us with a powerful choice. We have the opportunity to consume in a way that lightens the burden of global warming on the rest of the world.

Moving toward a more plant-based diet is also a way of voicing our resistance to a political system that denies human contributions to climate change and refuses to address it—something that challenges our standing in the world community. Will we imitate this failure to act in our own lives?

Although the threat of global warming is widely recognized, industrialized countries continue to fall short of making the kinds of meaningful changes that would slow it. Leaders in the United States have also failed to keep up with the rest of the world in even acknowledging the human cause and cost of climate change. But even those who express concern about climate change often avoid discussing changing one's diet for fear of alienating people. It's up to us to work with organizations that strive to protect the environment, engage in political resistance activities that push back against regressive policies, be in communication with elected representatives, and not be afraid to look at and change our own kitchen habits. Don't overlook the powerful impact of your food choices.

A plant-based diet is a way of voicing our resistance to a political system that denies climate change and refuses to address it.

Shrinking your personal carbon footprint isn't complicated. It's as simple as taking the beef out of your favorite chili and adding beans. Or trying a tofu scramble for breakfast. Or choosing the veggie burger—and some very delicious ones are now available—the next time you go out for a meal.

Daily Action 4:
EXPERIMENT WITH SOYFOODS

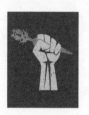

Soyfoods have a long history in Asian countries where they have been an important source of high-quality protein for centuries. The type and amount of soy in Asian diets varies by country and region, but generally people consume between one-half and two servings per day. The most common forms are tofu, soy milk, miso, edamame, and in Indonesia, tempeh.

As for all plant foods, soybeans use fewer natural resources and produce fewer greenhouse gases. What makes them special is that they are so rich in protein, providing more than other plant foods, even other beans. This means they are a particularly efficient protein delivery system.

They are also versatile, which makes them a fun addition to vegan diets. Here is a quick overview of the most commonly consumed soyfoods.

Edamame are green, immature soybeans, harvested at about 75 percent maturity. Unlike mature soybeans, they have a mild flavor. In Japan, they are a popular bar food, boiled in the pod and served with beer. You can find fresh and frozen edamame, shelled or in the pod. Boil them for 15 minutes in salted water and serve as a snack or an ingredient in grain salads.

Soy nuts are made from dry soybeans that are soaked and then roasted, sometimes with soy sauce or seasonings. They are an energy-rich snack, perfect for hikes, and are also a pleasant crunchy addition to salads.

Soy milk was an important part of Asian diets long before plant milks became popular in other countries. It's the liquid expressed from soaked, pureed soybeans. Use it to replace cow's milk in any recipe, to drink, or to pour over cereal.

Tofu is prepared by adding a curdling agent to soy milk. The curds are pressed into cakes of varying firmness. A slightly different process, but still using soy milk, produces a soft delicate product called silken tofu. In Asia, tofu is frequently served in soups or stir-fried with vegetables and rice or noodles. Vegetarians have discovered many nontraditional uses for tofu so that you find it now in puddings and custards, as a filling for lasagna, and in dips and sandwich spreads. Because its flavor is mild, it lends itself to all types of sweet and savory variations. It's impossible to do justice to tofu in just a few paragraphs; whole cookbooks are devoted to it. Once you start exploring tofu recipes, we're confident that you'll find ways to enjoy it.

Tempeh is an ancient culinary staple of Indonesia where it is still made in small home-based "factories." It's produced from whole soybeans, sometimes with rice or other grains added, which are treated with a starter and left to ferment, often wrapped in banana leaves in home preparation. The flavor is sometimes described as mushroom-like. It's especially good sautéed with vegetables and served over rice with spicy peanut sauce. It's also perfect to bake in barbecue sauce.

Miso, a salty, fermented soybean paste, is the essence of Japanese cooking. The variety and preparation of miso in Japan can be compared to winemaking in other parts of the world. It's used as a condiment to make broths and sauces and also makes a good replacement for parmesan cheese in pesto.

Textured vegetable protein, or TVP, is the frugal cook's friend. These dehydrated granules are made from defatted soy flour. TVP is low cost, packed with protein, and has a long shelf life. That's one reason you'll often find different types of flavored TVP in emergency food kits. Once it's rehydrated, it's often used to replace ground beef and particularly good in tomato-based dishes like chili, spaghetti sauce, and sloppy joes.

Here's the real news about soy and cancer: Soybeans are uniquely rich in plant chemicals called isoflavones. These compounds, also referred to as phytoestrogens or plant estrogens, can bind to the same hormone receptors in cells that the female hormone estrogen binds to. But the story about the biological effects of isoflavones is far more complex than this. They are actually selective in regard to which cell receptors they bind to, and the result is that they often have very different effects than estrogen in the body. In some cases they act like estrogen and in others they have antiestrogenic effects. Sometimes, they have no effects at all.

What we know from decades of research in humans is that soyfoods do not raise risk for breast cancer. In fact, evidence suggests that consuming soyfoods in childhood and adolescence can lower lifetime risk for breast cancer. Studies in both the United States and Asian countries find that women who have had breast cancer have a better prognosis if they are regular soy consumers. There is also evidence that eating soyfoods could lower risk for prostate cancer. Since high intakes of cow's milk have been linked to increased risk for prostate cancer, men would be wise to switch out cow's milk for milk made from soybeans.

DOES SOY CAUSE CANCER?

Soy Curls, which are made exclusively by Butler Foods in Oregon, are another dehydrated product, but they are made from the whole soybean. Soy curls are relatively new to the world of vegan cooking, but they have quickly gained legions of fans, particularly because of their pleasant chewy texture. If you'd like to try soy curls, we recommend also buying a jar of the company's Chik-Style Seasoning. Add a few tablespoons of the seasoning to the pan when sautéing the soy curls to create vegan chicken for soups, potpies, and stir-fries. Soy curls are also perfect for making a vegan version of bacon as you'll see in our recipe on page 65.

Tofu Corn Puffs

Makes approximately 24 bite-size croquettes

Light and fluffy, but with a rich flavor, these delicate little croquettes are easy to make and a good introduction for tofu skeptics. Make sure you use fresh bread crumbs, not dry. If nutritional yeast is new to you, see page 91 for a little more information about it.

2 slices whole-grain bread

½ cup cashews

½ cup water

½ pound tofu

¼ cup finely chopped onion

2 tablespoons nutritional yeast

2 cups corn (defrost first if using frozen)

½ teaspoon dried basil (or 1 tablespoon fresh chopped)

½ teaspoon salt

- Preheat oven to 350 degrees.

- Cut the bread into cubes and then pulse in a food processor to make bread crumbs. Set the bread crumbs aside.

- Place the cashews, water, and tofu in the food processor (you don't need to clean it out beforehand) and blend until smooth. Transfer to a bowl and mix in the rest of the ingredients.

- Use a melon baller or small ice-cream scoop to place croquettes on a nonstick pan. Spray the top of the balls with a mist of oil.

- Bake until set, about 20 minutes. Serve these as an appetizer or with a green salad and warm bread.

Five-Spice Baked Tofu

Makes 4 servings

Sometimes called Chinese Five-Spice, this seasoning is a blend of spices typically used in Asian cooking. It often contains cinnamon, star anise, cloves, hot pepper, and fennel, but there are many variations depending on region. The flavor of this dish will depend on which type of five-spice powder you buy, but it is always good!

1 pound firm tofu, drained
⅓ cup soy sauce
1 tablespoon water
1 tablespoon maple syrup (or any liquid sweetener)
1 teaspoon five-spice powder

- Cut the tofu into half-inch cubes and put these in a baking pan that is large enough to fit all of the tofu in one layer.

- In a separate bowl or measuring cup, combine the soy sauce, water, maple syrup, and spice powder. Pour this mixture over the tofu. Marinate in the refrigerator for at least one hour.

- Preheat the oven to 350 degrees.

- Cover the baking dish with foil and bake for 30 minutes. Uncover, stir the tofu, and then bake uncovered for an additional 20 minutes.

Edamame Hummus

Makes 2 cups

To make edamame hummus, simply replace the chickpeas in your favorite hummus recipe with cooked green soybeans. Here is our favorite way to make it.

¼ cup packed fresh parsley
½ cup tahini
¼ cup fresh lemon juice
2 cloves garlic, chopped
1½ cups cooked shelled edamame
Salt to taste

Place all ingredients in a food processor and blend until smooth. This hummus will keep in the refrigerator for 5 days.

Groovin' Reuben

Makes 4 sandwiches

Carol's son Ben used to make these all the time when he was in college and graduate school. One of his college friends, a nonvegan, declared it to be the best Reuben he ever tasted. Years later, he was still talking about this sandwich. We included it in our book *Never Too Late to Go Vegan*, and we use it here, too, because it is one of those recipes that, in its scrumptiousness, is perfect for all ages.

1 pound tempeh
3 tablespoons olive oil (more as needed)
3 tablespoons tamari (more as needed)
2 tablespoons water (more as needed)
1 cup sauerkraut
8 ounces vegan cheese (mozzarella variety works well)
Rye bread
Groovin' Reuben Dressing (recipe below)

- Steam the tempeh for 20 minutes in a steamer basket. Then slice it in half horizontally so that you have two thin slices. Cut each slice into four pieces.

- Stir together the olive oil, tamari, and water. Place the tempeh in a bowl and pour the marinade over it. Let the tempeh marinate in the refrigerator for an hour.

- Lift the tempeh out of the marinade and empty the marinade into a skillet. If all the marinade has been absorbed, mix together 1 tablespoon each of water, olive oil, and tamari and place in the pan.

- Heat the marinade over medium heat and add the tempeh. Cook covered between low and medium heat for 5 to 8 minutes. Turn the tempeh over, heap the sauerkraut on the tempeh, then top with the vegan cheese. Add a little water to the base of the pan, if needed, and cover, continuing to cook on low for 2 to 3 minutes until the cheese melts.

- Lightly toast the rye bread, spread the bread with the Groovin' Reuben Dressing, and add the tempeh smothered with sauerkraut and cheese.

Groovin' Reuben Dressing

Makes enough dressing for four Reubens

3 tablespoons vegan mayonnaise

2 tablespoons ketchup

2 tablespoons dill relish

1 teaspoon apple cider vinegar

¼ teaspoon salt

pinch black pepper

Combine all the ingredients, mixing thoroughly.

Daily Action 5:

LEARN TO LOVE LEGUMES

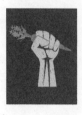

The family of legumes includes beans, soyfoods, and peanuts—all powerful sources of plant protein. Packed with nutrients and uniquely rich in both fiber and protein, they are linked to lower risk for many chronic diseases. Beans also lie at the heart of cuisines from all corners of the globe. And they are the most economical sources of nutrition of all foods, especially if you cook them yourself.

You can make beans in a pressure cooker, in a slow cooker, or on top of the stove. Soaking them overnight will speed up the cooking process, but for most beans it's not necessary. You may wish to soak chickpeas overnight, though, since they take a long time to cook. If you're sensitive to gas production from beans, soak them overnight and then discard the soaking water before cooking. This leaches out some of the sugars that may cause gas in some people.

To cook beans, rinse them well, place in a pot, and cover with four cups of water for each cup of beans. Add salt, bring to a boil, and then simmer the beans until soft. The cooked beans are ready to be used in any recipe you like. When you're in a hurry, canned beans are just as nutritious.

Beans lend themselves to all types of cuisine. You don't even need a recipe to turn cooked or canned beans into a fast meal. Here are seven ideas to get you started.

Main Dish Salad: Stir 1 cup of beans into 3 cups of any type of cooked grain. Add ¼ cup each of chopped onions and celery and dress with your favorite salad dressing and fresh herbs.

Mexican Beans: Stir ½ cup salsa and ½ cup corn into 2 cups of black, kidney, or pinto beans. Serve hot on a tortilla and top with avocado and chopped tomatoes.

Beany Sloppy Joes: Add a 15-ounce can of sloppy joe sauce to 2 cups of beans. Serve over toasted hamburger rolls.

Mediterranean Beans: Sauté ½ cup chopped onion and 3 minced garlic cloves in 2 tablespoons of olive oil. Stir in 2 cups of white beans and ¼ cup chopped roasted pepper or sun-dried tomatoes. Season with fresh herbs.

Barbecued Beans: Stir ¼ cup barbecue sauce into 1 cup of beans. Spoon over a baked potato.

Adzuki Beans in Miso Soup: Dissolve ¼ cup miso (see page 40) into 4 cups of water. Add one cup of cooked adzuki beans. Stir in ¼ cup sliced scallions just before serving.

Black Bean Dip: In a food processor, blend 1½ cups black beans, 1 tablespoon balsamic vinegar, ½ tablespoon fresh lime juice, 1 minced garlic clove, 1 tablespoon olive oil, ¼ cup chopped onion, and 1 table-spoon chopped fresh cilantro with salt and pepper to taste. Serve with raw vegetables or tortilla chips.

Baked Flatbread with Herbed White Beans

This bean spread can be made the day before, which will intensify the flavors. It also makes a delicious dip with raw vegetables or pita wedges.

Makes 4 servings as an appetizer

> 3 tablespoons extra-virgin olive oil, divided
> ¼ cup finely chopped onion
> ¼ cup finely chopped red bell pepper
> 3 garlic cloves, very finely chopped
> ½ teaspoon dried thyme
> ½ teaspoon finely chopped fresh rosemary
> 1½ cups cooked white beans (navy, cannellini, or great northern)
>   or one 15-ounce can

1 tablespoon fresh lemon juice

Salt and pepper

Large cooked flatbread or pizza crust

2 large tomatoes sliced

Fresh chopped parsley for garnish

- Preheat the oven to 400 degrees.

- Heat 2 tablespoons of the oil in a skillet and sauté the onion and
  red pepper until the onion is translucent, about 5 minutes. Add the
  garlic, thyme, and rosemary, and sauté for an additional minute.
  Add the beans and coat them with the oil and herbs. Turn off the
  heat and stir in the lemon juice. With a fork or potato masher, mash
  the beans to achieve a chunky texture. Season with salt and pepper.

- Brush the flatbread with the remaining tablespoon of olive oil.
  Spread the bean spread over the bread and top with the sliced tomatoes. Bake for 8 minutes until heated through. Sprinkle with the
  parsley before serving.

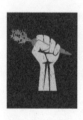

Daily Action 6:

TRY A VEGGIE BURGER

If it's available at an eatery near you, we highly recommend trying the
Impossible Burger. It recreates the precise flavors and textures, including
the red juiciness, of burgers made from beef, but from all-plant ingredients. Right now, the company that makes Impossible Burgers only
distributes to restaurants. For a similar experience in your own kitchen,
we recommend the Beyond Burger, found in the meat section or frozen
food section of many grocery stores.

You'll also find a wide selection of veggie burgers in the frozen
food section of almost any grocery store. Veggie burgers appear on the
menus of a growing list of restaurants, and you can find recipes for all
types of burgers made from combinations of beans, grains, vegetables,

and nuts. We've tasted burgers made with peanuts, beets, and even bananas. The sky's the limit when it comes to veggie burgers: They don't taste like hamburgers, and they aren't meant to. Homemade veggie burgers, like the one we share below, are delicious in their own right.

Smoky Black Bean Burgers

Makes 8 patties

Smoked paprika gives these black bean burgers their unique flavor. They are the creation of our friend Allison Rivers Samson, who specializes in healthy vegan comfort food. (You can find more information at her website: *www.allisonriverssamson.com*.) These burgers freeze well, so you may want to make a double batch. Serve them on hamburger buns with all your favorite condiments.

1½ teaspoons vegetable oil, plus more for sautéing the burgers
1 medium onion, finely diced
¾ cup celery, finely diced
4 cloves garlic, minced
1 teaspoon dried oregano
1 teaspoon dried thyme
1 tablespoon smoked paprika
¼ teaspoon chipotle chile flakes (optional)
3½ cups black beans, drained
1 teaspoon Dijon mustard
¾ teaspoon salt
½ teaspoon black pepper, freshly ground
1½ cups rolled oats (not instant)

• Heat 1½ teaspoons of oil in a large skillet over medium heat. Add the onion and sauté for 3 minutes. Add celery and sauté for an additional 2 minutes. Stir in garlic, oregano, thyme, paprika, and chipotle flakes (if using). Sauté for 2 more minutes. Remove from heat and set aside.

- In a large bowl, coarsely mash the black beans with a potato masher or the back of a fork. Stir in the mustard, salt, and pepper. Then, fold in the sautéed vegetables and oats and combine thoroughly.

- Line a large cookie sheet with parchment paper. Using a ½ cup measuring cup, portion 8 burgers onto the parchment paper and flatten to ½ inch thick.

- Lightly coat the skillet with vegetable oil and sauté the burgers over medium heat for 3 to 5 minutes or until browned. Flip the burgers and cook another 3 to 5 minutes until browned on the other side. Add oil as needed to keep burgers from sticking.

- Note: If you freeze your sautéed burger patties for later, let them thaw for 20 minutes before reheating. Heat them in the oven at 350 degrees for 20 minutes.

chapter 3

By the time the first Baltimore "Vegan Mac 'n Cheese Smackdown" competition overflowed its space in 2016, Brenda Sanders had been working in her community for several years on food justice issues. The mac and cheese competition was just another creative attempt to bring together many of the justice issues that concern her. "Mac and cheese is sacred in the black community," she told us. But, mac and cheese with no dairy? Yes, and it became its own delicious teaching moment. Brenda and her colleagues discovered this was yet another way to introduce their work of building a new food system within her community.

Brenda's activism addresses cruelty and inequities in food production and distribution. She creates innovative strategies to address the needs that arise from these inequities. One day finds her in a community garden. On another she is delivering vegan food to those who may not be able to access it otherwise. In addition to the mac and cheese competition, she is involved in running the Baltimore Vegan SoulFest.

Across the continent in California, another food justice activist, lauren Ornelas, is busy developing vegan Mexican recipes to combat what she calls "food apartheid": the imposition of white colonialist diets and foods, including dairy, on descendants of Mesoamericans. She is also working with migrant workers for safe living and work environments and running a school supply campaign for children of farmworkers. As part of the Food Empowerment Project, a nonprofit she founded in 2008 to address issues of food injustice, she develops reports on the lack of access to healthy foods in low-income communities of color. Her work is varied and far-reaching because that's the nature of food justice. Lauren says that working for food justice means looking "at the entire supply chain to make sure that all parties are treated with respect and given the opportunity to prosper and survive without suffering. And everybody has access to healthy and culturally appropriate foods."

Advancing food justice is complex, but efforts generally fall into four categories:

- Ensuring greater availability of healthy and culturally appropriate food.

- Working against food-driven climate change.

- Boycotting products that involve worker exploitation.

- Creating local, community-based, and community-informed solutions.

A vegan diet can be part of the response to these issues in several ways.

FOOD JUSTICE AND THE ENVIRONMENT

Rising sea levels, warming oceans, drought, and erratic weather challenge traditional livelihoods as well as food production as we talked about in chapter 2. While activists and nonprofits around the globe are addressing these issues, only a handful of organizations are considering the relationship of dietary choices to global warming and environmental destruction. One of these is the public policy action think tank Brighter Green. Executive director Mia McDonald and her colleagues work with community-based organizations, nongovernmental agencies, and individual leaders in Africa, Latin America, and developing countries in Asia to encourage policy action on issues that span the environment, animals, and sustainability. Brighter Green also engages directly in projects that seek to empower individuals and groups to create paths to sustainable development that mitigate the effects of climate change. Their work demonstrates the link between food justice and climate justice, showing how moving toward production of plant foods not only uses fewer resources, but also feeds people more healthfully and also has the potential to put food production under the control of marginalized populations.

According to Dawn Moncrief, who founded the Washington-based nonprofit A Well-Fed World, the world's least food-secure populations are also those disproportionately harmed by climate-related events, such as droughts, hurricanes, tsunamis, and flooding. These events don't just impact food production, but also food distribution, and create more opportunities for terrorism as we talked about in chapter 2. In a world where 20,000 people die every day from hunger-related diseases while wealthy populations overconsume meat, dairy, and eggs, the sources of which in turn overconsume land and other resources, Dawn's vision is one of a *well*-fed world. "A well-fed world is one in which everyone has enough food and the right kinds of food—that is, food that maximizes well-being for humans, animals, and the planet."

Environmental Racism

When animals graze in pastures, their manure is excreted onto the land where it recycles nutrients back into the soil. On today's factory farm, animals are crammed together in houses where their manure must be cleaned out and disposed of. The manure is usually stored in outdoor pits known as lagoons. There, it decomposes, emitting harmful gases. If flooding breaches the lagoons, contents can seep into waterways. This happened in 1999 in North Carolina when manure from pig farms spilled out of lagoons during Hurricane Floyd, leading to widespread water contamination.

In North Carolina, animals on hog farms produce nearly ten billion gallons of feces and urine. Some of the manure is transported out of the lagoons and sprayed back on fields, creating a filthy and stench-filled mist in the air. North Carolina is the second largest producer of meat from pigs in the United States, and its factory farms are located disproportionately near low-income communities of color. People living in these communities are at increased risk for illnesses associated with high levels of noxious gases such as asthma and food-borne illnesses. Exposure to chemical contaminants may be related to birth defects.

Unfortunately residents have little recourse. In many cases, relocating is not an option. And North Carolina lawmakers have put extensive limits on lawsuits against the farm owners. Waste from factory farms is a problem for everyone; manure from pig farms is an issue with environmental, health, and social justice dimensions.

FOOD INSECURITY

According to the U.S. Department of Agriculture, more than forty-one million people live in food-insecure households. This means that there are times during the year when households are unable to provide enough food for all family members. People may not have enough money to buy food, or they may lack other resources like transportation to purchase it.

Other factors affecting access may be more important, including affordability and also availability of food that is culturally appropriate. Calorie-rich unhealthy food is far more affordable than fresh fruits and vegetables. Foods like cow's milk, which many black and Hispanic people can't consume (see page 10), is considerably lower in cost, thanks to government subsidies, than almond and soy milk. In areas where McDonald's and 7-Eleven stores predominate but grocery stores are rare, people may have little exposure to alternatives to dairy.

The U.S. government defines a food desert as "a census tract that contains concentrations of low-income people in which at least a third of the population lives more than a mile from a supermarket or large grocery store. (For rural areas, the distance is 10 miles.)" Without a grocery store or supermarket, fresh food may be harder to obtain.

It's interesting that the term *food desert* relies on a description of a natural environment to describe a social environment created by social decisions. For instance, franchisees of the big fast-food corporations like KFC, Burger King, and McDonald's were able to get federal small business funding in the 1960s because each owner of a franchise was seen as a separate operator of the business. With federal support, multinational fast-food companies were able to move into the urban areas once avoided. National grocery retailers did not operate as franchises. Because corporations operated grocery stores, they were not eligible for the federal small business support and lacked the same incentives to bring their stores to the same areas.

The actual significance of food deserts is an issue of some debate. But, while research on this subject has been conflicting, prevailing opinion among public health professionals has been that lack of access to grocery stores, particularly when it is coupled with easy access to fast-food restaurants and convenience stores, translates to higher risk for chronic disease.

WORKERS AND FOOD JUSTICE

Slaughterhouse Workers

Food justice focuses not just on access but on those who work to bring food to the table. Early 20th-century writer and social activist Upton Sinclair spent six months investigating the Chicago meatpacking industry. His findings inspired his famous novel *The Jungle*, which followed the lives of Lithuanian immigrants working under shockingly inhumane and unsanitary conditions in a slaughterhouse. Allegedly, meat consumption fell by half after the book was published. The meat industry fought back. The Bureau of Animal Industry said that the allegations were "intentionally misleading and false" and "utter absurdity."

But due to public pressure, the federal government passed legislation aimed at ensuring adequate meat inspection, and it also established the government agency that eventually became the Food and Drug Administration.

Certainly, there were improvements, but one thing hasn't changed: More than one hundred years later, immigrants still suffer in dangerous conditions in slaughterhouses. As meat consumption has increased, line speed at slaughterhouses has increased in tandem. It's work that is physically demanding and requires the kind of repetitive motions that give rise to injuries. Workers might make ten thousand cuts over a single shift. Many suffer with chronic pain in their hands, wrists, arms, shoulders, and back. Rates of both injury and illness are unusually high among slaughterhouse workers. Repetitive motion, long hours, lack of time to sharpen knives, and pressure to increase speed combine to exacerbate risk of injury.

The psychological cost of this work is significant, too. According to a 2008 study in the *Georgetown Journal on Poverty Law & Policy* witnessing the pain and terror of the animals is very likely to produce psychological problems. Slaughterhouse workers may be susceptible to a form of post-traumatic stress disorder that occurs when someone participates in a situation that would cause them distress if they were the victim. It's called perpetration-induced stress disorder, and it can be linked to anger, violence, and domestic violence.

And so you might ask, "Who would want to do this work? Who wants to kill animals all day, every workday?" The answer, of course, is no one. And so the work is left to those who don't have a choice.

Slaughterhouse workers are predominantly people of color living in low-income communities, and about one-third are from Latin America. Often undocumented, non-English speakers, these are the most vulnerable workers who face occupational hazards and sexual harassment. Their undocumented status prevents them from reporting dangerous working environments or other violations of U.S. laws. Workers may fear losing their job or being deported if they seek medical care.

Along with undocumented workers, other vulnerable populations have been put to work in slaughterhouses. In South Dakota, Puerto Rican hurricane survivors began working in a turkey killing plant. It was called "a new answer in their ever-evolving struggle to find workers who would perform lower-rung American jobs." In rural Oklahoma, a "treatment program" for drug offenders that keeps them out of prison actually acts as a "labor camp" for slaughterhouses for large food companies. There they pull guts from slaughtered chickens that are purchased for fast-food restaurants and grocery stores, including Popeyes and Walmart. They receive no actual treatments, nor do they receive their own wages, which go instead to Christian Alcoholics & Addicts in Recovery.

Perhaps the most invisible group of workers is the largely immigrant workforce who cleans up the slaughterhouses after the stunning, shocking, killing, skinning, gutting, deboning, chopping, breast-pulling, toenail-cutting, bird-hanging, and other interventions with the bodies of dead animals occur. With their disinfectants and scalding water, they scour the place, removing fragments of bodies and the blood. Injuries inevitably occur.

Exploitation of this lower-rung labor force helps keep meat prices down in the supermarket. Other food justice issues exist in food production, especially the labor and exploitation of farmworkers, but the treatment of those who kill and those who clean up after the killing is a central issue for food justice.

Chocolate Bars and Child Slavery

What could seem more cozy and benign than a cup of hot chocolate on a cold winter evening? What's more fun than sneaking a few candy bars from your kids' Halloween stash? But the production of much of the world's chocolate involves the exploitation of children. Cacao farmers in West Africa earn less than $2 per day, and to keep their costs low, they often use child labor. Children working on these farms may have been sold by their impoverished families or abducted by traffickers. They work long days in extraordinarily dangerous conditions, involving heavy knives, machetes, and even chain saws. They may live in unsanitary conditions with inadequate food. They may be beaten if they try to escape or work too slowly. In the Ivory Coast, 40 percent of children who work on cacao farms don't attend school.

Conditions vary among cacao farms, but nearly two million children in Ghana and the Ivory Coast work under the worst forms of child labor. The large companies that profit from the $60-billion chocolate industry could help these children simply by paying cacao farmers a living wage that would allow them to produce cocoa without slave labor and child labor.

Unfortunately, it's difficult to know if the chocolate you buy was produced with child labor, and labels like "fair trade" aren't standardized for candy. Generally speaking, chocolate sourced from West Africa is very likely to involve child labor or slave labor. The Food Empowerment Project offers a list of chocolates that are both vegan and ethically sourced. They offer free apps for both iPhone and Androids so you can easily make an informed purchase the next time you head to the grocery store.

HEALTHY FOOD FOR ALL

Brenda Sanders's activism began when she learned of the shocking twenty-year difference in life expectancy between populations living in white affluent sections of Baltimore and poor black areas. While there were many factors responsible for the differences, diet and chronic disease were clearly significant ones. Brenda bought food demo equipment and carried it from church to church and from health fair to health fair, educating people about ways to eat a more plant-based diet. She confronted the injustice of the lack of options for the people she was teaching and notes the racist perspectives that give rise to that injustice. Brenda says that too many people "think that 'these poor black and brown people don't care.' They *do* care; they want something different but it's not in their reach. Once we come in and say, 'do you want this?' they say they do."

> **Everyone, no matter their economic status, should have the option to be vegan.**

Everyone, no matter their economic status, should have the option to be vegan and the chance to make choices that are more sustainable and aren't harmful to animals. It is racist to assume that people living in marginalized communities can't experience empathy and compassion or that they aren't trying to solve the problem when, in fact, they often weren't being given the consideration or the funding.

Community gardens are an effective way to promote food justice. They bring healthy, affordable, and culturally appropriate foods to people who may have limited access to these foods. In Baltimore, people flock to these gardens, Brenda says. "Kids, families—it was magical. We created a sanctuary of sorts in these urban communities. Once you build a garden, the insects come and the birds come. The kids had never seen a red bird, a praying mantis. The kids were so impressed seeing all these animals in the 'hood.' And the parents were given a chance to connect to the kids."

Urban gardens can indeed be transformative, as efforts in Milwaukee, Wisconsin, also show. In this Rust Belt city of 600,000 people, there are more than 150 urban gardens and 26 farmers' markets, making it the city with the highest number of gardens per resident in the United States. Residents are allowed to sell the produce they grow at farm stands and markets. The local Victory Garden Initiative provides a raised bed, seeds, and gardening lessons to anyone who wants to try their hand at gardening. The group aims to create a "socially just, environmentally sustainable, nutritious food system for all." It's not a trendy "food movement," though, according to Venice Williams, the executive director of another organization called Alice's Garden. "There's nothing I'm doing that my family hasn't done for generations," Williams, who is of African American and Choctaw descent, says. Among those who are finding that urban gardens can help them gain their footing in a new community are Milwaukee's Syrian refugees, some of whom come from farming backgrounds.

Every time you choose a vegan meal, you're creating space for justice.

Over the years, grassroots activists have sometimes seen their efforts turn into something with far greater impact than they ever dreamed. In 1974, the seeds of the nonprofit Plenty International were sown when members of a vegan farm community in Summertown, Tennessee, started giving away their crop surpluses to local people. Since those early days of distributing vegan food to impoverished local communities, volunteers have fanned out across the United States and also to countries in Central America, the Caribbean, and Africa. Dubbed "The Hippie Peace Corps," the organization teaches food production skills, improves nutrition through protein-rich plant foods, brings books to low-income children, and provides health care and disaster relief.

Food Not Bombs (FNB) was also founded by a handful of activists nearly forty years ago. Beginning in 1980, volunteers gathered to protest war and poverty and to share free food. With a focus on justice for both humans and farmed animals, FNB chapters distribute only vegetarian food (they strongly encourage vegan options) and are involved in community antipoverty, antiwar, and pro-immigrant organizing. Volunteers also provide food to protesters and striking workers and organize food relief after natural disasters. Today, there are chapters in nearly 500 cities in countries in Europe, the Middle East, Africa, the Americas, Asia, and the Pacific region.

A newer, but rapidly growing organization that addresses hunger relief through vegan meals is Chilis on Wheels. Local chapters distribute hot vegan meals to people who are homeless or living with food insecurity. Volunteers also provide dog food for dogs living with homeless people.

CREATING FOOD JUSTICE IN YOUR KITCHEN

You may not be in a position to start a community garden or a local hunger relief group, but there are things you can do that have a meaningful impact on fighting food injustice. Choosing more vegan foods is a start. It reduces your contribution to global warming and boycotts products that exploit slaughterhouse workers. It also represents an important shift in the way most people think about food. That is, when you start exploring all the impacts of a vegan diet, it becomes clear that eating is an act that is about far more than personal health or pleasure. Looking at the impact of vegan food choices on others, both humans and animals, creates space for food justice. Many vegans have discovered that their new appreciation for the power of food choices has led them to become more involved in local food justice efforts.

As we've seen in this chapter, there are also opportunities to address food justice that go beyond veganism. Expand your commitment to the #GrabYourWallet campaign by choosing to buy chocolate that doesn't exploit children. Or make a commitment to avoid restaurants that exploit their workers with guidance from the ROC National Diners Guide (a guide on the working conditions of American restaurants from the Restaurant Opportunities Centers). We also recommend the YEI Food Justice App developed by teens with the Youth Empowerment Project to teach their peers about food justice. Or bring vegan food to hungry people. (See Daily Action 10.)

Consider ways in which you can share ideas about food justice within your own social circles. If you are a member of a church, start a campaign that says, "The best mission trip you can take is to become vegan," that focuses on issues of food justice. The next time you contribute something to a bake sale fundraiser, consider brownies that are labeled as "Vegan and Ethically Sourced Chocolate" as a way of starting conversations about these issues. Find ways to share food with people who live with food insecurity.

And, of course, every time you choose a vegan meal, you're creating space for justice for slaughterhouse workers, justice for animals, and justice for the environment.

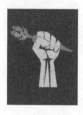

Daily Action 7:

TRY A VEGAN MACARONI AND CHEESE RECIPE

You don't need dairy cheese for this comfort food; make a dish that's inclusive and delicious.

Carol's Mac and Cheese

Serves 8–12

This is Carol's adaptation of a very rich recipe that included three kinds of cheeses and two kinds of milk. When she serves it at her yearly Fourth of July vegan barbecue, everyone comes back for seconds—and thirds!

For a slightly less rich recipe, halve the vegan mozzarella and cheddar. Serve at your barbecue or on its own.

½ pound elbow macaroni or mini penne, precooked and drained
½ to 1 cup cashews (soaked overnight if you do not have a high-
    speed blender)
1½ cups water
1 14-ounce can coconut milk
8 to 10 ounces of silken tofu
1 teaspoon Dijon mustard
4 cloves garlic
½ teaspoon turmeric
¼ to ½ teaspoon cayenne
¼ to ½ teaspoon paprika
½ teaspoon salt
Freshly ground black pepper to taste
1 head of kale, washed, destemmed, and shredded or a bag or
    two of baby kale
1 bag vegan shredded mozzarella cheese
1 bag vegan shredded cheddar cheese
½ cup nutritional yeast

- Prepare the macaroni or penne. After draining it, place in a large mixing bowl.

- Blend the cashews with the 1½ cups of water.

- Add the coconut milk, silken tofu, Dijon mustard, garlic, spices, salt and pepper into the blender and thoroughly blend together.

- Mix the blender ingredients with the cooked pasta.

- Add the shredded or baby kale (lots!), the two bags of cheese, and the nutritional yeast.

- Spray the bottom and sides of the inside of a slow cooker with non-stick vegetable spray.

- Put the macaroni and cheese mixture into the slow cooker. If you were tempted to add more than 8 ounces of macaroni, add some unsweetened soy milk if the mac and cheese looks too dry.

- Cover and cook on high for 60–90 minutes. Then turn to low until the mac and cheese solidifies, at least three more hours. It is okay if some of it sticks to the sides.

Daily Action 8:

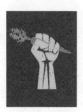

TRY A VEGAN VERSION OF BACON

Removing bacon and other meat from pigs from your menus is a way to protect the earth and to support both the people and animals who are victims of factory farms.

Vegan Bacon

Commercial plant-based bacon is available for vegans who miss the salty, smoky flavor of these foods. Look for Sweet Earth Hickory & Sage Smoked Seitan Bacon, Lightlife Smart Bacon, Tofurky Smoky Maple Bacon Marinated Tempeh, and Upton Naturals Bacon Seitan.

If you need something to sprinkle on a salad, Betty Crocker Baco-s Bits and McCormick Bac'n Pieces are vegan. For sautéing greens or making biscuits, Vegan Magic, made with coconut oil, is an alternative to bacon grease.

These products are fast and convenient, but it's also fun to make your own bacon. You'll find recipes for bacon made from soy curls, rice paper (really!), tofu, tempeh, seitan, eggplant, and mushrooms.

One essential ingredient for making vegan bacon is liquid smoke, which you can usually find in the spice section of the grocery store. According to Bryanna Clark Grogan in her cookbook *World Vegan Feast*, liquid smoke is made by channeling smoke from smoldering wood chips through a condenser. This causes the vapors to liquefy, trapping the water-soluble flavor compounds in the liquid. All of the nonsoluble compounds are filtered out, leaving behind a safe and clean way to give dishes an appealing smoky flavor. You'll find that many vegan bacon recipes rely on some combination of liquid smoke, salt, and a sweetener to achieve bacon-like flavor.

Soy Curl Bacon

Serves 6

Chewy soy curls flavored with smoked paprika and liquid smoke are a satisfying alternative to bacon. If you can't find soy curls in any local stores, order them directly from Butler Foods or any of the online vegan groceries in the resource section on page 183. You can also use tempeh in place of the soy curls.

½ 8-ounce bag soy curls
2 tablespoons maple syrup or any liquid sweetener
3 tablespoons soy sauce
1 teaspoon smoked paprika
2 teaspoons liquid smoke
2 tablespoons vegetable oil

- Place the soy curls in a heatproof bowl and cover with boiling water. Let this stand until the soy curls are soft, about 10 minutes. Drain and press to remove any excess water.

- In a separate bowl combine the maple syrup, soy sauce, smoked paprika, and liquid smoke. Pour this mixture over the soy curls. Let the curls marinate in the refrigerator for at least an hour.

- Heat the oil over medium heat and add the soy curls with their marinade liquid. Sauté until browned.

- Serve on toasted bread with lettuce, tomato, and vegan mayonnaise.

- If you are using tempeh, steam 8 ounces of tempeh for 10 minutes and then slice into thin slices. Marinate for an hour and sauté.

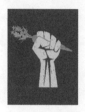

Daily Action 9:

BAKE WITH ETHICALLY SOURCED CHOCOLATE

Download the Food Empowerment Project's chocolate list before heading to the store. Or check the website for a list of ethically sourced chocolate: *www.foodispower.org/chocolate-list*.

Zucchini Brownies

Makes 12 brownies

These are moist and chewy—like a brownie should be! The addition of baby food prunes makes them incredibly moist and rich.

    2 cups flour
    1½ cups sugar
    1 teaspoon salt
    1 teaspoon baking soda
    ½ cup unsweetened cocoa powder
    2 tablespoons vanilla
    ¼ cup oil
    ¼ cup pureed baby food prunes
    2 cups peeled and grated zucchini
    ½ cup walnuts (optional)

- Preheat the oven to 350 degrees. Grease a 9-by-13-inch pan.

- Combine the flour, sugar, salt, baking soda, and cocoa in a bowl. (If your cocoa tends to clump, sift these ingredients together.)

- Add the vanilla, oil, prunes, zucchini, and walnuts (if you are using). Mix well. This may take a while as the zucchini releases a little moisture!

- Pour mixture into the greased pan and bake. Check at 30 minutes, though it may take just a few minutes longer.

- Optional: sift some confectioners' sugar on top.

SIGN UP TO HELP BRING VEGAN FOOD TO HUNGRY PEOPLE

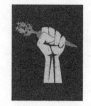

Efforts to get healthy plant foods to hungry people are growing in major cities and even small towns. Check the websites to see if there is a Food Not Bombs or Chilis on Wheels group near you or to get help in starting one.

Another way to help get healthy plant foods to hungry people is to donate to your local food pantry. Canned beans, TVP, pasta, spaghetti sauce, and shelf-stable packages of fortified plant milks are all good choices.

Best Vegan Chili

Makes 6 servings

This has been the go-to vegan chili recipe in Ginny's family for years. It's also a perfect recipe to make in bulk to distribute outdoors to anyone who needs a hot meal. It tastes even better when reheated the next day.

    1 cup boiling water
    1 cup dry TVP (see page 40)
    2 15-ounce cans diced tomatoes
    1 8-ounce can tomato sauce
    1 large onion, coarsely chopped
    1 green bell pepper, chopped
    1 teaspoon cayenne powder

2 tablespoons chili powder (or to taste)

2 teaspoons cumin powder

2 teaspoons garlic powder

1 teaspoon dried oregano

¼ teaspoon allspice

1 15-ounce can kidney, pinto, or black beans

- Pour the boiling water over the TVP and let this sit for 5 minutes.

- Combine with remaining ingredients except the beans in a sauce-pan, cover, and simmer for one hour.

- Add the beans and simmer for an additional 30 minutes. Serve in bowls with corn bread.

chapter 4

TAKE OUT MISOGYNY

Animal agriculture is a major vehicle for maintaining and disseminating misogynist attitudes. It may not seem obvious at first, because so many of the practices are hidden from view. But there could be no meat, dairy, or eggs without continuous sexual exploitation. Farmers keep female animals pregnant until they are killed. The ongoing reproductive exploitation that undergirds animal agriculture requires a misogynistic view of females and of female reproduction.

We are going to show you in this chapter how the oppression of farmed animals strengthens misogyny. There is misogyny not just in the way these animals are treated but also in the way farmers, pharmaceutical companies, and farmworkers talk about them. We are also going to look at how attitudes toward meat consumption contribute to viewing females as objects and are expressed through advertisements. This "take out" misogyny goes all out. It crosses over from women to female animals and back again, deliberately playing with and collapsing female identities with a wink that attempts to disarm its harms while reinforcing hateful attitudes.

One aspect of misogyny is the equation of women with their bodies. Bodily functions like pregnancy, lactation, and menstruation are seen as animallike and have long been viewed as processes that undermine rationality, making women appear biologically closer to animals than men. Misogyny is an engine that drives unequal status and treatment. This inequality has been insinuated within laws, practices, and institutions in ways that empower men and disempower women and those equated with women. Whether it is expressed through practices that affect the lives of women or the lives of animals, it serves to uphold the patriarchal order. Even if it is hidden from most of us, it has repercussions for all of us.

MEAT AND MASCULINITY

In Carol's book, *The Sexual Politics of Meat*, she argued that meat and masculinity have become linked, expressed in the assumption that men need to eat meat to enhance their masculinity. Conversely, failure to eat meat threatens this masculinity, as does a preference for eating vegetables, which are the domain of the feminine. Contemporary expressions of these beliefs are easy to find. A *Muscle and Fitness* magazine cover shows a well-muscled, shirtless white man thrusting a piece of raw meat toward the viewer while stabbing another piece of meat with his other hand; "Eat Like a Man," the headline proclaims. Male-identified settings such as steak houses, fraternities, strip clubs, and barbecues promise both male bonding and meat, guaranteeing an unchallenged freedom of consumption. A *Boston Globe* review of a steak house referred to its fare as "testosterone wrapped in bacon."

Advertisements for fast-food businesses beat this idea into the ground. Chicken platters are called "Man Platters." A video for Taco Bell's "Triple Steak Stack" features "Hurricane Doug," who learns a steak dish "three times the size" is "what a man eats."

It's not just about selling food. In a Hummer commercial, a man buying tofu at a grocery store is suddenly overcome with anxiety when he sees another man's cart filled with red meat. The tofu-buying man runs to the nearest dealership to buy a Hummer. The original tagline for the short video advertisement said, "Restore your manhood." It was later changed to "Restore your balance."

In all of these ads, meat eating becomes a marker—*this* is what real men do; they eat meat. They aren't "sissies"; they aren't "effeminate." They won't eat food identified with women and equated with "weakness." There is an irony in all this: equating meat with freedom and strength requires accepting anxious cultural dictates about maleness while being afraid to challenge stereotypes about gender. It also requires a willingness to benefit from cowardly ways of raising, traumatizing, and killing animals.

This perceived link between meat eating and attributes of strength and freedom has been embraced by white male supremacists who have originated the term *soy boy* to insult liberal men. Drawing on the popular and incorrect belief that soy raises estrogen levels in men, it implies

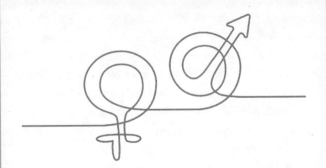

The term soy boy reflects the unfounded belief that eating soy results in higher estrogen levels, lower testosterone, and feminine traits in men.

It's not difficult to see where these beliefs come from. Soybeans are uniquely rich in isoflavones, a type of phytoestrogen or plant estrogen. But these isoflavones are not the same as the female hormone estrogen.

In humans, soy isoflavones had harmful effects on male hormone status only in a couple of cases where men consumed absurdly large amounts of soy—more than twelve servings per day.

Clinical research on soy and male hormones paints a much more reassuring picture. More than forty studies, including those in which men consumed higher amounts of isoflavones than is typical in Asia, showed that regular consumption of soy isoflavones does not impact testosterone levels, sperm count, or sperm quality. For guidance on how much soy is safe to eat, it's helpful to look at traditional consumption patterns throughout Asia, where the average is about one-half to two servings per day and some men eat as much as three or four servings.

liberal men are less likely to eat meat, rendering them "weak" and "womanlike." The masculine-fetishized right-wing views the moniker as a devastating insult. Soy boy is a reminder that what people eat carries political meaning.

SEXUALIZING ANIMALS

Meat advertisements suggest that animals desire their fate as edible, using images and language to represent this desire as sexual. In doing so, the advertisements manufacture a framework that legitimates viewing women (and animals) as sexually consumable. Many of these advertisements compare a woman's body to dead, consumable animals, use stereotypes of women's sexual availability to mask animal suffering, and leverage femaleness as the ultimate insult. This is a tool that reaches into homes, greets drivers via billboards, circulates in social media via memes, and is as powerful as other media that dismiss sexual harassment and glorify sexual exploitation.

For instance, a Chicago restaurant featured the "Double D Cup Breast of Turkey Sandwich" on its menu. "This sandwich is SO big," the menu boasted, giving men permission to joke about women's breasts. (What you won't see on the menu is why the breasts are so big. Turkeys are bred for such large breasts that they can't walk to be slaughtered; they topple over.) In California, Rosie the *Original* Organic Chicken poses in red high heels, necklace, and hat proclaiming her "organic" nature to consumers. The images announce that she wants you to consume her. A visit to Portland, Oregon, could have brought you face to face with an advertisement for a "hot chicken" shack. There she stands, in her high heels, stockings, and a bustier, posing

> **Rosie the *Original* Organic Chicken poses in red high heels, necklace, and hat . . . the images announce that she wants you to consume her.**

seductively, her eyes meeting yours. "Come and get me," she invites. "Come and *eat* me," she means.

These ads do not just use stereotypes of women's sexual availability to advertise meat. They also suggest that farmed animals actually in bondage are "free," free in the way that "sexy" women have been depicted as free, sexually available as though their only desire is for the viewer to want their bodies.

We tend to gloss over the ways in which feminized animals contribute to the degradation of women. "It's just a chicken image, for goodness' sake!" Or "it's just a menu item." In fact, it is far more insidious than that.

Sexualized and edible body parts do not have a voice.

Well before the 2016 presidential election, a popular anti–Hillary Clinton political pin read: "KFC Hillary Special: 2 Fat Thighs, 2 small breasts . . . left wing." Former Australian prime minister Julia Gillard was the subject of a similar attack when the opposition party held a dinner that included on its menu "Julia Gillard Kentucky Fried Quail: small breasts, huge thighs and a big red box."

Two of the most powerful women in the world have been reduced to sexualized and edible body parts. The political discourse reflects an actual advertisement from Kentucky Fried Chicken that asks, "Are you a breast man or a leg man?" Substituting a body part for an entire person takes the idea of women as objects a step further. This fragmentation might make it hard to acknowledge the harm; but the harm is disempowerment: the whole woman has disappeared, and sexualized and edible body parts do not have a voice.

MEAT ADVERTISEMENTS SUPPORT RAPE CULTURE

One of the challenges for prosecuting rapists is that consent is determined from the point of view of the rapist not the rape victim. There is a parallel here with meat eating. Meat-eaters like to believe their victims have consented to their deaths, often describing it as "a sacrifice" made by the animal. Consider a popular internet meme that renames chicken parmesan as "chicken permission." Next to a photo of the menu item a living chicken is depicted saying, "Yeah, ok, sure go ahead." A sign for The Saussie Pig BBQ in Florida advertises a cartoon image of a pig balanced on heels, wearing red garters and a leotard, beneath the words "Moanin' for the Bone." What about the delivery van in New Zealand with white-stenciled letters on its side window, "Warning! Hot Chicks Inside"?

These examples of meat advertisements operate in tandem with the fiction of consent in a rape culture. They make meat eating appear playful and harmless. They depict defeated females who desire their defeat. This desire for death and their own consumption is framed according to traditional assumptions about female sexual desire to be overpowered.

"Breastaurants" take the "playfulness" to a new level—offering actual women to ogle in meat-centric environments. Even the names of these establishments—Hooters or Twin Peaks, for example—are double entendres that create an impression of permission for overt sexual harassment while encouraging fantasies of consumption. "Better Grab a Pair," Twin Peaks tantalizes.

Restaurants, advertising, and male meat culture offer permission to view females as desirous of exploitation and consumption. This is misogyny. What is not so obvious, what is hidden from the consumer, is that many of the animal products we consume are dependent upon the continuous exploitation of female bodies and female reproduction. This has become take out misogyny.

REPRODUCTIVE EXPLOITATION ON THE FARM

One in five women in the United States have visited Planned Parenthood for health care. Women depend on this organization to take control of their reproductive health. When this control is taken out of their hands, an absence of respect for women's bodily integrity pervades.

Most of us do not realize it, but a conversation about female sexual availability and reproductive control has been going on for decades, unobserved by the average person. Animal agriculture could not exist if it didn't control female bodies and reproductive cycles. Without the constant pregnancy of female animals, there could be no meat, milk, or eggs for human consumption. If misogyny nests in attitudes about meat consumption, it's given free rein in the attitudes of animal agriculture toward reproduction. After all, to control and enhance fertility one must have absolute access to the female of the species.

Even within the industry, advertisements aimed at farmers often deliberately confuse to whom this control of reproduction is refer-ring—women or other female animals. Drug companies depict sexy, buxom females who *want* to be made pregnant, who *want* to give the farmers more babies each year, who *want* to "pump out baby pigs." A cartoon pig named Lisa is shown in stockings, heels, garters, and lip-stick as she fondles her medicine. The ad promises "Lisa gives you one more pig per year." The ad implies, Lisa *wants* to give you one more pig per year. But it's a safe bet that Lisa does not want to produce baby pigs on a factory farm. Kept in gestation crates and then farrowing crates, sows in captive reproduction are prevented from expressing their maternal instinct, which is to nurse and care for their piglets away from humans.

On dairy farms, cows wear ear tags with their numbers. In a promi-nent Facebook discussion group for farmers, when one posted a photo of a cow with the ear tag "bitch from hell," others quickly chimed in about how delighted they are to send their cows to slaughter when they "misbehave" [read: resist]. Absolute power, abuse of the female, sexual exploitation—so of course, she's become a "bitch."

A pharmaceutical company advises farmers: "Keep your cows preg-nant and on the job." In fact, pregnant or not, a dairy cow is nearly always "on the job." She produces milk several times a day and calves every year to ensure that milk production continues. When it doesn't, she's still on the job and becomes hamburger.

Toward the end of 2017, Dairy Air, a liquid nitrogen ice cream shop opened in New Jersey. Its logo featured the backside of a heavily sexualized cow, so that if you hadn't caught the double entendre with *derriere*, you can't miss it once you encounter the logo. The cow has pouty lips, lidded eyes, and her tail is lifted off her plump rump as if she were ready for you to forcibly impregnate her. (Once customers get past the logo and are inside the store, they are greeted with ice cream flavors like Backside Banana Split, Sweet Cheeks and Chocolate, Spankin' Strawberry Moon, and Muffin-Top Money Maker.)

As with her sisters depicted through oppressive images, it is not dignity that is conveyed, but desire. The Dairy Air cow *wants* to be held captive and impregnated. The website wikiHow provides an explanation of how to artificially inseminate "the Female Bovine": "First, position the cow in a captive position so she is immobilized and cannot protest, for instance in a squeeze chute."

What is interesting is that animal agriculture denies that this treatment of cows and chickens is even *sex*, much less *violent*. Animal studies fellow Kathryn Gillespie of Wesleyan University observes: "There is all this work to obscure the fact that it is not sexualized violence, not violence, not sex, yet looking at the [bull] semen industry, a lot of their advertising materials—the t-shirts, boxer shorts, mugs, and other paraphernalia they sell—reveal through humorous puns and jokes about the process that it is an act of sex, it is an act of sexual violence."

Dr. Gillespie points to an advertisement from a cattle semen company. "[It] pictures a grinning cartoon bull, two lipsticked cows in the background spreading their hind legs and presenting their backsides, and the slogan, 'We Stand Behind Every Cow We Service.'"

Ecofeminist writer and activist pattrice jones is the cofounder of VINE Sanctuary in Springfield, Vermont, an LGBTQ-run farmed animal sanctuary. Her work has given her the opportunity to extensively study the life of cows. She says, "Whatever word you use for this, it's forced penetration by a foreign object of an immobilized female, and at least part of the purpose is an expression of power and control."

How Sexual Violence Myths Function Toward Female Animals

For years, we have heard the same myths defending sexual violence against women. There are stark comparisons to how animal agriculture defends the sexual violation and reproductive coercion in dairy and egg farming.

She wanted it.
On the farm: *The female cow wants to be forcibly entered and made pregnant.*

She deserved it.
On the farm: *She's a bitch from hell.*

She liked it.
On the farm: *She needs us to take her milk* and *only happy hens lay eggs.*

Women are the weaker sex; they need protection.
On the farm: *Animals are safer when they are confined; it protects them from other animals and the elements. It keeps them from trampling their babies.*

FACT: *Just as the home is a very unsafe place for victims of marital rape, incest, and domestic violence, the farm is a place where frightened, abused, and physically overused animals live and die.*

On factory farms, animals have no power to resist this forced penetration. In a natural environment, a cow can position herself to be mounted or she can simply walk away if she so chooses. Cows cannot walk away from their imprisonment in the animal agriculture industry.

"LIVESTOCK": HOW MISOGYNY BLURS THE LINES

What appears to be a feature of life, misogyny, is actually a one-sided construct, a particular point of view arising from and perpetuating entitlement. The same kind of entitlement that undergirds animal agriculture and fuels popular cultural depictions of animals who will be eaten as female is expressed in attitudes toward women who have suffered sexual exploitation.

In early 2018 Cornell University made headlines with a story that was a stark example of the blurred lines between attitudes toward women and attitudes toward animals. Cornell's Zeta Beta Tau fraternity was placed on a two-year probation after members were found engaging in a contest called a "pig roast." In the secret game, members earned points for having sex with large women. In the event of a tie, the member who had sex with the heaviest woman won. The competition targeted and degraded women, especially large women, by viewing them as objects and as animals. It wasn't invented at Cornell, though. Instead, it's a long-standing practice on campuses that aims to humiliate and demean women. Traditionally, it goes by the name "hogging." Not a single individual who initiated it or participated in it at Cornell was expelled.

In turning a kaleidoscope, the light and the fragments remain the same though they align differently, presenting changing colors and shapes. It's the same for misogyny in our culture; while the assumptions and attitudes remain the same, they find different vehicles for expression: playing with ideas of sexual availability; comparing a woman's body to dead, consumable animals; using stereotypes of women's sexual availability to mask animals' suffering while affirming

No one wants to be forced to reproduce or fulfill someone's fantasies as a piece of meat waiting to be consumed.

the legitimacy of the original oppressive image; leveraging femaleness as the ultimate insult while assuming something about gender and food consumption; reducing women to their body parts and equating them with pieces of meat; *and* making women's reproductive health decisions the domain of men.

Women's rights to self-determination are undermined by reproductive control of nonhuman females. And the idea that female animals might also possess bodily integrity slips even further from ethical consideration when women's rights to reproductive care are restricted. This relationship is perhaps best summarized in a 2013 meme from Democrats Organizing for America. It was responding to a punitive and restrictive abortion law and featured a picture of a cow next to the question: "What do you call a female who is not allowed to control her own reproduction?" The answer was "LIVESTOCK." Some mistook it as a pro-animal rights message. It was not. It was comparing women to cows only to sound the alarm on behalf of women's rights.

RESISTING MISOGYNY

Although all animal agriculture is built around exploitation of female reproduction, the practices are most obvious and unceasing on hog, egg, and dairy farms. Female animals are forced to spend their lives producing babies, milk, and eggs solely for human consumption. They do so until they are too worn out or sick to be profitable. Then they are sent to slaughter. These are the lives of female farmed animals whether owned by families or corporations. It is true whether these foods are produced by conventional methods or when they are organically produced.

There is often a "which came first, the chicken or the egg?" aspect to discussions of misogyny. Which came first, an understanding of female reproduction that led first to the domestication of animals and then the oppression of women? Or did the oppression of women occur without this aspect of control of fertility and reproduction?

Ten thousand years later, many of us have opinions on this. Some well-respected scholars even suggest that all of human oppression builds on the oppression of animals. But we don't need to trace back to the beginnings to recognize how we can work against misogyny. We march with our "pussy hats," protect abortion clinics, support Planned Parenthood and use their services, and call attention to forced sterilization. We work to elect more pro-choice women at all levels of government. We challenge sexual harassment and exploitation and seek accountability for the abusers.

We can also look past the species barrier and acknowledge that no one wants to be forced to reproduce or fulfill someone's fantasies as a piece of meat waiting to be consumed.

Daily Action 11:
MAKE VEGAN CHEESE

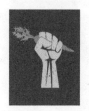

Commercial vegan cheeses, often made from nuts, coconut, or soy, just keep getting better but it's also surprisingly easy to make your own. We offer a couple of options here to get your feet wet. Cashew cheese makes a good filling for lasagna or to spread on crostini for a party. We also offer a quick tofu feta to use as a spread or in a traditional Greek salad.

Crostini with Cashew Cream and Tapenade

Makes 20 appetizers

The soft cashew cream in this recipe gets depth from the use of miso, a salty fermented soybean paste we talk about on page 40. Be sure to soak the cashews beforehand or you'll end up with a grainy cheese.

2 tablespoons extra-virgin olive oil, plus more for brushing bread
½ cup chopped sweet onions
1 cup raw cashews soaked overnight
1 tablespoon miso
1½ tablespoons fresh lemon juice
1 loaf French bread
½ cup tapenade (any type)
Chopped fresh parsley for garnish

- Preheat the oven to 425 degrees.

- Heat the oil and sauté the onions until translucent.

- While onions are cooking, drain the cashews and process in a food processor or high-speed blender until creamy. Add the sautéed onions, miso, and lemon juice, and process to combine the ingredients.

- Slice the bread into ½-inch slices. Brush with olive oil on both sides and place in a single layer on a baking sheet. Bake until crisp, about 6 to 8 minutes, turning once.

- Spread each bread slice with the cashew cream and top with about a teaspoon of tapenade. Sprinkle with chopped parsley.

Greek Salad with Vegan Feta

It's easy to create some of your favorite dishes without depending on your own form of take out misogyny by using some vegan feta!

Serves 4–6

- 1 red onion, thinly sliced
- 1 head crisp Romaine lettuce, chopped
- 1 cup vegan feta cheese
- 1 medium cucumber, peeled, halved lengthwise, and sliced and sprinkled with salt and pepper
- 1 6-ounce jar marinated artichoke hearts
- 1 red bell pepper, sliced
- ½ fennel, thinly sliced
- 1½ cups cherry tomatoes
- ½ pound Greek olives
- 1 15-ounce can garbanzo beans, drained and rinsed
- ⅓ cup parsley, coarsely chopped
- 1 avocado, peeled, sliced

For dressing for lettuce:

- 4 tablespoons olive oil
- 2 tablespoons freshly squeezed lemon juice
- 4 teaspoons balsamic vinegar
- ½ teaspoon salt
- ½ teaspoon fresh ground black pepper

For dressing for red onion:

- ⅛ cup red wine vinegar
- ½ teaspoon salt
- ½ teaspoon organic granulated sugar

- Place the red onions in a bowl. Bring the red wine vinegar, salt, and sugar to a boil. Remove from heat and pour over the onions. Place the onions in the refrigerator to cool for at least an hour.

- Combine the ingredients for the lettuce dressing in a jar and shake. Add this mixture a tablespoon at a time to the chopped lettuce and toss. It should be very lightly covered.

- Arrange the lettuce to cover a large oblong or round platter. Arrange the onion on the outer perimeter of the lettuce. Place the feta cheese in the middle of the platter. Arrange the cucumber, artichoke hearts, sliced peppers, fennel, tomatoes, and olives around the cheese. Sprinkle the garbanzo beans and parsley over the whole platter. Just before serving, slice the avocado and arrange on the platter.

Tofu Feta

Makes 2½ cups

Vegan cream cheese and plenty of salt give this vegan cheese the flavors and richness of feta. You can also spread this on French bread for an appetizer. Or reduce the salt to 1 teaspoon and use to replace ricotta cheese in stuffed shells.

1 pound extra-firm tofu
4 ounces nondairy cream cheese of your choice, softened to room
    temperature
¼ cup extra-virgin olive oil
¼ cup fresh lemon juice
1½ teaspoons salt
½ teaspoon garlic powder

- Rinse the tofu and pat it dry with paper towels. With your hands, crumble it into a bowl.

- Mix in the cream cheese, oil, lemon juice, salt, and garlic powder. Store in the refrigerator for up to a week.

Daily Action 12:

REPLACE EGGS IN SAVORY OR SWEET RECIPES

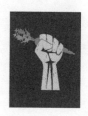

It's easy to veganize common favorites like egg salad sandwiches and scrambled eggs with the addition of just a few ingredients.

Scrambled Tofu

Serves 4

Having a good tofu scramble recipe to draw upon and alter at will depending on the ingredients in your refrigerator can be a mainstay for a quick, easy meal. Scrambled tofu is versatile! You could add steamed broccoli, chopped potatoes, green peppers, vegan bacon—well, you get the idea. Brunches with scrambled tofu are always a hit. The turmeric in this recipe gives the tofu the color of eggs.

> 1 tablespoon olive oil
> 3 garlic cloves, minced
> 8 to 10 medium mushrooms, sliced
> ½ cup carrots, grated
> ½ cup scallion
> 1 pound regular firm tofu, crumbled
> 3 tablespoons nutritional yeast
> ¼ teaspoon turmeric
> 1 tablespoon soy sauce
> 1 cup spinach, baby kale, arugula, or chard
> 2 avocadoes (optional)

- Heat the oil over medium-high heat, then sauté the garlic and mushrooms until they are golden on one side. Flip the mushrooms and add the carrots and scallion. Sauté for about 2 minutes.

- Add the tofu, nutritional yeast, turmeric, and soy sauce. Stir and continue cooking for about 5 minutes.

- Add the greens, cover, and let cook for about 1 minute so they become slightly wilted.

- Serve with one-half avocado sliced onto each plate, if desired.

- Note: If you plan to add any other ingredients or cooked vegetables to your scramble, do that before adding the greens.

Eggless Salad with Black Salt

Makes 4 sandwiches

Black salt, also called Himalayan black salt or *kala namak*, is a type of rock salt found mostly in the Himalayas. It smells and tastes remarkably like hard-boiled eggs due to its sulfur content, making it a valuable addition to your pantry for recreating egg salad or other dishes that use eggs. Black salt is actually pink in color, but it's not the same as the product called pink salt. Be sure to look specifically for *kala namak*. You may need to scout it out online since it's typically sold only in specialty grocery stores.

Most eggless salad recipes use tofu, but we love this interesting idea adapted from a recipe on the vegannomnoms.net website and originally from a German vegan cookbook. It uses chickpeas plus macaroni. The pureed chickpeas provide a consistency similar to egg yolks while the macaroni provides a texture similar to cooked egg whites. Make sure the macaroni is cooked well; it should not be al dente.

1 cup cooked chickpeas

1 teaspoon vegetable oil

2 cups cooked elbow macaroni (or any type of small pasta)

½ cup vegan mayo

¾ teaspoon black salt or to taste

- Puree the chickpeas and the oil in a food processor.

- Scrape the chickpea puree into a bowl and put the noodles into the food processor. You don't need to clean it out first since you'll be combining everything anyway. Process just until the macaroni is cut into small bits.

- Add the macaroni bits to the chickpea puree and mix in the vegan mayonnaise. Season with the black salt, adjusting the amount according to your taste.

- Variation: If you can't find black salt, you can still turn this recipe into a delicious filling for sandwiches. Follow the directions above, but add 2 teaspoons yellow mustard, 6 sliced scallions (white and green parts), 4 sliced celery hearts, and ½ tablespoon vinegar. Let the mix refrigerate for two hours to allow the flavors to meld.

Replacing Eggs in Baking

Vegans who like treats find plenty of ways to indulge their sweet tooth. You can browse the internet to find recipes or give a few tweaks to some of your family favorites to make them vegan. It's true that some desserts present a little bit of a challenge. For example, we've not yet seen a reasonable vegan version of an angel food cake, with its twelve egg whites. But any cake or cookie recipe that calls for just one or two eggs can easily be made vegan with the aid of egg replacers.

Here are a few of the most popular egg replacers for baking:

Commercial Egg Replacer Powder: Usually made from some combination of starch ingredients and leavening agents, these powders are added directly to the recipe with the addition of a specific amount of water (usually 3 tablespoons) to replace each egg.

Flaxseed: Combine 1 tablespoon of flaxseed powder with 3 tablespoons of water and mix well. Let stand for 10 minutes until the mixture thickens to a consistency like egg whites. This egg replacer is most useful for pancakes, muffins, or brownies. It's not effective in some cake recipes.

Soy flour: Add one heaping tablespoon of soy flour plus two tablespoons of water for each egg. Soy flour can help make eggless cakes fluffier and lighter.

Aquafaba: Derived from Latin for "water" and "bean," aquafaba is made from liquid left over from cooking beans, usually chickpeas. It is all the rage in vegan baking these days. Simply drain the liquid from a can of chickpeas. For baking, aquafaba should be the consistency of raw egg whites. If it's too thin, you can thicken it by simmering over low heat until it cooks down to the right consistency. Replace each egg (up to 3 per recipe) with 3 tablespoons of aquafaba. Or use 2 tablespoons to replace an egg white. Aquafaba can even be whipped to form stiff peaks if you'd like to make a vegan meringue. If cooking with aquafaba intrigues you, we highly recommend the Aquafaba (Vegan Meringue - Hits and Misses!) group on Facebook. With more than 80,000 members, you'll be in good company as you explore recipes and tips using aquafaba.

Crazy Cake

Serves 9

Families were snacking on this vegan cake before the word *vegan* even entered our language. It dates back to the Depression and was especially popular during World War II when eggs were being rationed. It gets its lightness from the action of baking soda and vinegar.

    1½ cups all-purpose flour
    ¼ cup unsweetened cocoa powder
    1 cup white sugar
    1 teaspoon baking soda

½ teaspoon salt

1 cup water

5 tablespoons vegetable oil

1 tablespoon white or cider vinegar

1 teaspoon pure vanilla extract

- Preheat the oven to 350 degrees.

- Stir together the flour, cocoa, sugar, baking soda, and salt.

- Combine the water, oil, vinegar, and vanilla in a large measuring cup. Pour over the dry ingredients and mix by hand just enough to combine thoroughly.

- Pour into an 8-inch square or round cake pan.

- Bake on middle rack of oven for 35 minutes. Check with toothpick to make sure it comes out clean.

Frosting for Crazy Cake

6 tablespoons vegan butter, softened

1½ teaspoons vanilla

$2\frac{2}{3}$ cups confectioners' sugar

½ cup unsweetened cocoa powder

$\frac{1}{3}$ cup plant milk

- Place the butter and vanilla in a bowl and beat until creamy. Add the sugar and cocoa, mixing well. Add the milk in two additions, mixing each time.

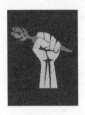

Daily Action 13:

INVITE PLANT-BASED UMAMI INTO YOUR LIFE

"I could go vegan, but I just can't give up cheese" is a comment we hear often. But the cravings we associate with cheese are often a craving for something else altogether. What people are missing is most likely *umami*. The word is derived from the Japanese term for "deliciousness," and it's been dubbed the "fifth taste" (in addition to sweet, sour, bitter, and salty). Umami was discovered more than one hundred years ago by a Japanese researcher. It's a sort of taste/experience/essence in foods that is imparted by high levels of the amino acid glutamate.

One theory about the appeal of umami is that, because breast milk is high in glutamate, we might develop a lifelong desire for this taste beginning within hours after birth. Aged cheeses are especially high in umami, and this may be why they are so compelling. But it's not at all difficult to add umami to vegan meals. Fermented foods have umami, so wine, tamari, and miso are good additions to dishes. Ripe tomatoes are loaded with umami and so are concentrated tomato products like ketchup, tomato paste, and sun-dried tomatoes.

Marmite, nutritional yeast, mushrooms, olives, balsamic vinegar, dried mushrooms, and sauerkraut are other umami-rich vegan foods. Sea vegetables are rich in it; in fact, umami was originally discovered in kelp. Roasting, caramelizing, browning, and grilling are cooking techniques that impart umami flavors.

If you are someone who just feels you could never give up cheese, try experimenting with these umami-rich ingredients. You may find it's easier than you think.

VEGAN CHEESE

Vegan cheese has come a long way in the past couple of decades. If you remember it as something that refused to melt and tasted like plastic, it's time to get reacquainted with all of the wonderful new products on the market. Not only are there several choices for making a grilled cheese sandwich, but cultured artisan vegan cheeses—usually made from nuts—mean that you can throw a fun wine and cheese party, vegan style.

Faux Parm

Makes ½ cup

This recipe is a little bit of a miracle. It includes just three ingredients and takes about three minutes to make. The result is a topping for pasta, beans, rice, or vegetables that takes flavor instantly to the next level. In addition to making any savory dish taste wonderful, faux parm provides essential omega-3 fats from the walnuts, vitamin B12 from the nutritional yeast, and iodine from the salt. It's packed with umami thanks to the nutritional yeast (lovingly referred to as "nooch" by many vegans). If you're allergic to nuts, you can substitute sunflower seeds.

½ cup walnut halves
3 tablespoons nutritional yeast
1 teaspoon iodized salt

- Pulse the walnuts in a food processor until very finely ground.

- Add the nutritional yeast and salt and give it another few pulses to mix everything thoroughly.

- Store in the refrigerator. It can also be frozen.

chapter 5

DREAMING OF AN INCLUSIVE DEMOCRACY

HOW SOCIAL OPPRESSION RELIES ON ANIMALITY

Animality is a potent weapon when used to disempower individuals, ethnic groups, and races. It refers to a quality or nature associated with animals. When *human* and *animal* are viewed as opposites, animality becomes a potential slur against humans and, as such, a tool for social oppression. It also offers oppression an alibi, allowing us to exclude any beings deemed "animals" from moral consideration. In this way, social oppression leverages animality against targeted groups of humans and uses that association to justify their disenfranchisement.

White racists often label African Americans as animals, specifically as primates. Recent examples include depictions of President Barack Obama as an ape and Michelle Obama as an "ape in heels." A racial discrimination lawsuit against Texaco charged that blacks were called "orangutans" and "porch monkeys" in the workplace. Alabama legislators who sponsored a bill aimed at suppressing the black vote were caught on tape referring to black voters as "aborigines" and "illiterates." Calling out to Ferguson, Missouri, demonstrators following the death of Michael Brown, an unarmed eighteen-year-old black man killed by police, one cop yelled, "Bring it, all you f—king animals." Following the death of Freddie Gray at the hands of the police, Baltimore County police officer Jennifer Lynne Silver referred on Instagram to protestors as "animals" and a "disgrace to the human race."

RACE IS A HOAX AND ANIMALITY IS PART OF ITS DECEPTION

Race is a hoax. So writes Kevin Young in *Bunk: The Rise of Hoaxes, Humbug, Plagiarists, Phonies, Post-Facts, and Fake News*. Race is a hoax because it is a classification that changes meanings and definitions over time. For instance, before the Civil War, when large parts of the United States allowed the enslavement of an entire race, racial definitions at times were flexible. Southern racial laws and legal opinions determined whiteness by a formula of fractions. In Virginia, for example, persons who were one-eighth black were legally white. Someone could also be considered "white by reputation in the community." After the Civil War, those customs fell by the wayside and were replaced by the "one-drop rule." One drop of black blood, one distant black ancestor, made an individual black.

Definitions change and so, too, do characterizations of races. During slavery blacks were often depicted as children needing to be guided or controlled by a benevolent white. After slavery, the image of blacks, especially black men, changed to a dangerous animal, a beast needing to be hunted down and destroyed. Blacks were said to be degenerating, moving downward, regressing from civilization.

> **When *human* and *animal* are viewed as opposites, animality becomes a potential slur against humans and, as such, a tool for social oppression.**

The hoax of race requires elaborate explanations, which have also changed over the centuries. Once many Christians believed that blacks descended from Ham, who was cursed by his father Noah. Then, pseudoscientific claims displaced religious explanations. For example, 19th-century Harvard scientist Louis Agassiz proposed that the races were created separately. Known as "polygenesis" it was a theory of largely U.S. origin, used to argue that certain groups were inferior and to justify slavery.

Race-making relies on the human-animal dualism. Jason Hannan, a rhetoric scholar at the University of Winnipeg, refers to that "group of racist terms used by the voices of European imperialism to justify power and domination over non-European peoples, terms like 'savage,' 'primitive,' 'wild,' 'uncivilized,' and 'barbaric.' These terms connote not only cultural difference, but also cultural inferiority, evoking the image of 'wild' animals in a state of nature. 'They' are categorically different from 'us,' because they stand outside the realm of culture and civilization altogether. They therefore need to be tamed and civilized by the cool hand of European power."

Characterizations of African Americans as more animallike than whites subtly endure. We see this in advertisements that depict African Americans not only as athletes, but feature them as successful athletes in sports associated with force, like boxing or football, rather than with noncontact sports associated with intellectual skills. This is part of the anomaly of golfer Tiger Woods and the late tennis champion Arthur Ashe.

Race-making needs animals to help demarcate who is a citizen and who is not. The animal is primitive, uncivilized, without dignity; humans—citizens!—are advanced, civilized, possessors of dignity. The failed businessman huckster who hoaxed himself into the U.S. presidency gained political attention in 2011 by asking for President Obama's birth certificate. It was a dog whistle to his racist followers who chose to believe that the first black president was not a U.S. citizen. Within the explicit racism of the demand for the birth certificate something deeper and more harmful was implied: Trump, white = citizen, versus Obama, not "American," African (Kenya) born = subhuman, animallike.

The claim was outrageous, but it didn't matter. Disaffected whites hitched their racist aspirations and beliefs to an orange-haired white man. But something sinister about Trump's beliefs about his followers is also revealed. With these dog whistles, his followers, too, are animalized: It's not just that they can hear and respond to something that others can't—like a dog answering to a high-pitched sound. It's that a dog whistle also *trains* a dog.

ANIMALITY AND DISEMPOWERMENT

What is the quality of being an "animal" that *animality* exploits? Humans have long underestimated animals, who, like the crow who makes tools, the octopus who defends herself with rocks, and the dog who nurses orphaned kittens, continue to surprise us with their abilities and sensibilities. The debate is no longer whether animals have consciousness but what kinds?

We use animality against animals all the time by flattening their diversity into stereotypes, failing to recognize their cognitive abilities, and denying their social nature and social affiliations. Birds can grasp abstract concepts and are now considered "feathered apes" because of their cognitive processing skills. But "birdbrained" remains an insult. Pigs are as smart as dogs, yet "pig" remains a negative term when used about humans. We deprive animals of freedom of movement, freedom to take care of their young, and of their own lives, and then say they have no autonomy. Studying animals and marine life without the blinders of dominant attitudes, we encounter the immense diversity on the other side of the species line: fish that change sex, animals who choose same-sex relationships and have cross-species friendships, and other evidence that animals do not offer a mirror to oppressive viewpoints about sexuality and gender.

> **The debate is no longer whether animals have consciousness but what kinds.**

Animality keeps us from identifying with or sympathizing with other animals. It also keeps us from identifying with or sympathizing with other humans when we animalize them or view them as less than human. It throws them toward the species border, justifying and perpetuating forms of domination. Tainted by animality, their claims to be citizens are contested.

WHO'S A CITIZEN?

There has always been a human/animal binary aspect to racist, misogynistic, and ableist logic. In the political sphere, animality functions as a tool for democratic exclusion. Oppression elevates some humans as deserving equal protection and equal participation as citizens and lowers others, by making them "other" and suggesting they are more like animals.

From the beginning of U.S. history, the concept of *citizen* excluded many. The founders marked white, male, property owners as "citizens" with rights. Assumptions about who was a citizen were embedded within a very narrow understanding of who was a *human*. To have status as a citizen with full participatory rights in the democracy, you had to be seen as possessing human qualities rather than animallike qualities.. White male democracy was built on exclusion.

In the 19th century, "mere adult white maleness" replaced 18th-century requirements for citizenship. You didn't even have to be a taxpayer. This was known as "universal suffrage" even though it was not at all universal. Adult white male suffrage made the United States, in the words of Nell Painter Irvin "a white man's country."

As they worked for their enfranchisement in the 19th century, some white middle-class women allowed animality to function on their behalf. They sought to parse the Constitution to include them but exclude others. They claimed, to paraphrase them, "We aren't the animals. We are the pure. We are the educated. We aren't the dirty immigrant, the illiterate freed slave." Always, in debate over who was a citizen and who was not, animality influenced the conversation. Like a barnacle clinging to the side of ship, it is difficult to remove it once it has attached itself. At times, the pitting of the disenfranchised against each other causes us to fail to confront the common problem—the roots of democracy based on exclusion and its limited notion of a citizen.

RACE IS A HOAX AND AUTONOMY IS A FICTION

The men who wrote the Constitution in the United States and the Declaration of Rights and the Citizen in France were deeply influenced by the Enlightenment and perspectives on the autonomous person. *Autonomy* means acting independently, but it's also usually perceived as meaning "able to be self-sufficient."

The idea that anyone is truly independent and acting autonomously is a fiction, influenced by racist, misogynist, and ableist stereotypes. We first learn essential skills such as walking and talking from others. The "self-made man" benefits from an entire hidden or rarely acknowledged support system including most often a wife and secretary and sometimes servants. Stephanie Coontz says that "Self-reliance and independence worked for *men* because *women* took care of dependence and obligation. The cult of the Self-Made Man required the cult of the True Woman."

Donald Trump actively exploited the fiction of self-sufficiency during the presidential campaign of 2016. Despite his birth into wealth, the assistance his father provided, the nameless staff that enabled his work, the tax benefits he leveraged, the ghostwriter for his book, Trump cultivated the idea that he succeeded on his own, a self-made man. He also benefited from generous subsidies from banks.

In *Beasts of Burden,* Sunaura Taylor points out that one result of this prizing of "independence" is that disabled people's lives are often seen as tragic. But, dependence is relative, according to British disability activist Michael Oliver. People with disabilities see independence as the ability to be in control of and make decisions about their own lives, rather than being able to dress, wash, or cook without help.

Lawrence Carter-Long, communications director for the Disability Rights Education and Defense Fund, reminds us that part of the criterion for inclusion is how useful a person is to a society. He notes disabled people are often compared to animals to evoke their dependency and supposed limitations. Terms used to demean intellectually disabled people (which also demean animals) include birdbrained, harebrained, cuckoo, lamebrained.

Taylor points to the ways in which dependency has been used to justify slavery, patriarchy, colonization, and disability oppression. "The language of dependency is a brilliant rhetorical tool, allowing those who use it to sound compassionate and caring while continuing to exploit those that they are supposedly concerned about."

But, we are all vulnerable and will all need care at some point in our lives. Our dependency goes well beyond the need for acute care. Most

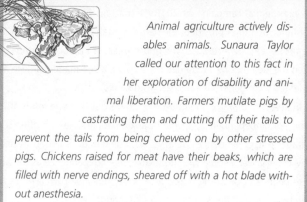

DISABLING ANIMALS

Animal agriculture actively disables animals. Sunaura Taylor called our attention to this fact in her exploration of disability and animal liberation. Farmers mutilate pigs by castrating them and cutting off their tails to prevent the tails from being chewed on by other stressed pigs. Chickens raised for meat have their beaks, which are filled with nerve endings, sheared off with a hot blade without anesthesia.

Lameness is a common affliction across species as animals are bred to grow too quickly and may be forced to stand without relief on wire-mesh, concrete-slab, and metal-slat floors in their confinement buildings. One report has estimated 50 percent of pigs are lame at the time of slaughter. Cows are bred to produce excessively large quantities of milk. Many become lame because the size of their udders strains their hips or forces their back legs apart.

of us are dependent on a huge support network that provides us with fuel, water, food, and home maintenance. We rely on wild animals to maintain the integrity and balance of the natural world. And while we see domestic animals as dependent on us, their dependency is something humans have imposed upon them. We have done so in violent ways to extract their labor or their flesh for food.

WHO IS A TERRORIST?

Throughout the past few decades, white supremacist groups have grown in the United States. Yet, during that time, two groups have been the focus of federal enforcement: Muslims and animal rights/environmental activists.

Since 1990, the Southern Poverty Law Center has tracked hate groups (917 in the United States as of this writing) and radical, anti-government militias. During that same time, federal resources were directed toward labeling sabotage and property damage as terrorism and prosecuting as terrorists those who used those tactics—animal and environmental activists.

In 2004, the deputy assistant director of counterterrorism for the FBI reported, "The FBI's investigation of animal rights extremists and eco-terrorism matters . . . [It] is our highest domestic terrorism investigation priority." The FBI also said that in "the three years following 9/11, every act of domestic terrorism, except for one, was the work of animal rights and environmental activists."

White supremacy groups and antigovernmental right-wing militias were growing, as well as attacks on abortion clinics and the murder of doctors who performed abortions, but no corporate pressure existed to stop them—they were not affecting anyone's bottom line the way animal rights activists and environmentalists were (see pp. 16–17).

Targeting animal rights activism in the 21st century echoes similarly skewed priorities of the 1950s. At a time when both local police and the FBI went to extraordinary lengths to infiltrate and disrupt left-wing political groups, hound gays and lesbians working in the government, and investigate organized crime syndicates, they largely ignored a nationwide terror campaign against African Americans who integrated white communities.

When we consider the vast majority of those who have murdered multiple individuals—white supremacists attacking African Americans, Jewish, Latinx, and Muslim citizens; antiabortionists killing medical doctors; homophobes and transphobes killing LGBTQIA people; and husbands who exterminate their entire family—one common characteristic prevails: most are white men.

Still our idea of "terrorists" is of brown-skinned individuals or those "extremists," eco-terrorists. Instead of being seen as terrorists, those white men who stockpile arsenals and kill their family or groups of strangers are called "lone wolves." This helps us to interpret home-grown white terrorist violence as an anomaly. The failure to label these men as terrorists reveals the resilience of the dominant conceptualization about who is a citizen—still, the white man—and who is not. It shows, as well, the danger of holding to a prevailing stereotype that favors one group of citizens. Activists are labeled terrorists, and terrorists, the everyday kind, the ones shooting up campuses and churches are not; they are "lone wolves," perhaps the one group that benefits from its association with animality, even though it sorely misrepresents wolves.

THE ARC OF THE UNIVERSE

We live with a deeply held myth of historical progress. This myth holds that there has been an ongoing improvement in living conditions; that over the centuries, rights have expanded and tolerance has grown. The expectation is that we will continue to move forward, albeit slowly as "the arc of the moral universe is long, but it bends toward justice."

There are two major problems with this myth. One is that the arc of justice has not been consistently moving forward. The second is that this myth of political progress may prevent us from recognizing the erosion of democratic institutions.

Underneath the myth of political progress we find evidence that progress has repeatedly been undercut and democratic principles betrayed by a devolution in rights. Settler colonialism destroyed Native foodways, introduced the diet of beef-loving English people, exposed Native peoples to diseases they were not resistant to, perpetrated the murder of millions, and also robbed Native American nations of land. At the same time, the lives of indigenous people were erased from history. Memorials and markers of "first" sites usually refer to those that are relevant to white history: "first" town, "first" settlement, "first" dwelling.

In 1877, federal troops were withdrawn from the former Confederate states ending "America's first experiment with interracial democracy after the Civil War." With this withdrawal, black entry into the civic world was reversed, Reconstruction ended, and an unchecked reign of terror accompanied the adoption of Jim Crow laws. The period gave rise to memorials to treasonous whites who fought for the South during the Civil War and a suppression of black efforts at memory-keeping that centered on Emancipation. A full century later, in the 21st century, we are still debating the presence of these memorials. At the same time, emancipated slaves and their descendants were forced into involuntary servitude, a type of "slavery by another name," as journalist Douglas A. Blackmon called it. This human labor trafficking supplied workers to brick factories, coal mines, lumber camps, and local white farmers.

In the 21st century, black men have been targeted through the War on Drugs, so that 40 percent of the incarcerated population is African American, while African Americans only make up 13 percent of the population. The U.S. criminal justice system has become a new operator for racial control which Michelle Alexander calls *The New Jim Crow*. The criminal justice system, after labeling people of color "criminals," then enables the denial of certain privileges of citizenship. For example, in some states felons are not allowed to vote until they have completed parole and reregistered. In others, the governor of the state must restore their voting rights.

Nor has justice moved steadily forward for other groups. We continue to see ongoing encroachments on abortion rights, efforts to deny civil rights to transgender individuals, assault on same-sex marriages, and, of course, fear-mongering about both terrorism and the economy aimed at banning new immigrants and expelling those who are already here.

And while those in power work tirelessly to turn back the clock on human rights progress, the dog whistle heard by some convinces them that they are victims, returning the focus to the original "citizen."

Vegans know about fictions of progress. They inform some of the most deeply held justifications of eating meat and dairy: that humans are at the top of the food chain, that we are the evolutionary victors and entitled to the spoils of that victory, which are animals' bodies. A popular bumper sticker asserts, "I didn't get to the top of the food chain to be a vegetarian."

Focusing on how different animals are from us allows us to use them as we want.

You might think that vegans spend their time interrogating ingredient labels, looking for the stray whey and the unneeded egg. But what we have learned to interrogate is the propaganda that encourages meat, dairy, and egg consumption. It comes from corporate advertising and with the full backing of the federal government.

Animal activists could point out how Western meat eating became coupled with this faith in political progress and democratic optimism. The four food groups of the 1950s were tied to two myths that interweave: that meat provides the best form of protein and the myth of cultural (and culinary) improvement—that our diet is constantly improving. Yet, it is hard to imagine that the arc of the universe bending to justice includes usurping one-third of the landmass of the world to be used for animal agriculture. Or that it bends toward justice when we are slaughtering more animals than ever and confining them in worse ways than ever.

Faith in political progress may keep us from recognizing the erosion of democratic protections and systems. If we believe that basic democratic institutions can withstand any assaults, we may miss the signs that they are instead crumbling. Timothy Snyder, a historian of modern Europe at Yale University, says that the optimistic assumption that the federal government can withstand assault on its institutions may prevent us from responding accurately and fully.

We see worrisome assaults on freedom and democracy in countries throughout the world, among them the autocratic tendencies introduced by Donald Trump and embraced by some segments of the U.S. population. These include depicting the mainstream press as unreliable, offering alternative false narratives, undercutting regulatory control, gutting government institutions, showing a weak commitment to democratic rules, demonstrating a willingness to curb civil liberties, toleration or support of violence, and using federal law enforcement agencies to go after an administration's opponents—not to mention a troubling fondness for and praise of other authoritarian leaders. In response, our protests must be broadly based, vigorous, and not only *against,* but *in* defense of rights and institutions.

SOCIAL JUSTICE ADVOCACY: WHAT DO WE DO ABOUT ANIMALITY?

If the way to keep those viewed as different and undesirable is a process of dehumanizing through animalizing, where does that leave the animals? We can stop animalizing other humans, pulling them away from the barrier that divides us from nonhuman animals, but that still leaves animals sitting solidly on the other side of that line. To say, "We *aren't* animals" as an argument for respect and inclusion sanctions animality as a force for exclusion.

Abolishing that line, as far as treatment and protection go, is essential to eliminating the effects of animalization on humans. One reason animality makes for such a potent resource for social oppression is because all around us is proof of how easy it is to debase the animal, especially in agriculture, but also in entertainment and research. Focusing on how different animals are from us allows us to use them as we want.

Even though we often forget it, we humans are animals, too. Like us, the other animals are capable of feeling fear and pain and loneliness and sorrow. We recognize that humans differ from one another, but the similarities eclipse the differences when it comes to basic rights and treatment—at least in theory. Likewise, we can seek to learn more about commonalities among species while celebrating differences. For, if we are so different from the other animals, what does our humanity ask of us in our treatment of them? And if we are like animals, as we are in so many ways, what does our shared animality ask of us?

The arc of the universe needs our help to bend toward justice.

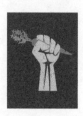

Daily Action 14:

PACK YOUR FREEZER WITH SNACKS FOR PROTEST DAYS

Whether it's an all-day march at the nation's capital or a quick lunchtime protest right in your own town, resisting burns calories. Keep your freezer packed with homemade energy bars that you can slip into your pocket. We've also included a recipe for rosemary-infused nuts, which make a good on-the-go snack. And don't forget about peanut butter sandwiches when you need a grab-and-go snack. Peanut butter has a long history in U.S. vegetarian cuisine. It was invented in 1895 by John Harvey Kellogg to replace meat in the diets of patients at his sanitarium in Battle Creek, Michigan. It's packed with energy and protein, making it a perfect choice for long days of protest. Pair it with slices of bananas or

apples, with shredded carrots, pickles, or jelly. If you're allergic to peanuts, choose almond, cashew, hazelnut, pumpkin, or sunflower seed
butters instead. Spread on crackers, bagels, English muffins, or whole-
grain breads, and you'll be ready for a long day of resistance work.

Peanut-Butter Oat Energy Balls

Makes 24 balls

Keep these no-bake energy balls in the refrigerator or freezer for on-
the-go snacks. This recipe is fun to make with children and allows for
plenty of flexibility. Use any combination of nut or seed butter, chopped
nuts or seeds, and dried fruit you prefer.

> 2 cups quick oats
> ½ cup ground flaxseed or toasted wheat germ
> ¼ cup sliced almonds
> ¾ cup chopped apricots
> ½ teaspoon cinnamon
> 1 cup smooth natural peanut butter
> ½ cup maple syrup or any liquid sweetener

- In a large bowl, stir together the oats, flaxseed, almonds, apricots,
  and cinnamon.

- Place the peanut butter and sweetener in a small saucepan and heat
  over low heat just until the peanut butter is melted. Pour this mixture over the dry ingredients and combine thoroughly.

- Form the mixture into walnut-size balls and place on a cookie sheet.
  Put in the refrigerator for at least an hour to cool. You can also press
  these into a 9-by-13-inch baking pan, refrigerate, and then slice into
  bars.

Rosemary Nut Snacks

Makes 8 servings

These are based on a recipe that appeared in the *Dallas Morning News*. Carol revised it to create a vegan snack that is lower in salt and sugar than the original.

> 2 cups raw unsalted nuts of your choice (Try a mix of walnuts, pecans, and almonds.)
> 2 tablespoons vegan butter
> 3 tablespoons light brown sugar
> 3 tablespoons chopped fresh rosemary
> ½ teaspoon kosher salt

- Preheat the oven to 350 degrees.

- Spread the nuts on a baking sheet in a single layer, and roast for 10 minutes.

- While nuts are roasting, melt the butter. Stir in the sugar, rosemary, and salt.

- Transfer the nuts to a bowl, add the butter mixture, and mix with a wooden spoon. Spread the nuts back onto the baking sheet and allow to cool.

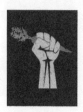

Daily Action 15:

MAKE A GREENS AND BEANS BOWL

If anything can bring people together, it just might be greens and beans. This powerful duo appears on tables in some form or another throughout the world. Combine any type of bean with spinach, kale, collards, mustard greens, bok choy—whatever you prefer. Flavor with sautéed garlic and onion and any herbs or spices you like.

Simple Stewed Pinto Beans and Collard Greens with Tahini Drizzle

Serves 6

This recipe comes to us from nutrition expert and inspired vegan cook Gena Hamshaw. The tahini drizzle takes a very simple dish to the next level. We highly recommend Gena's blog *thefullhelping.com* for more cooking inspiration.

1 tablespoon olive oil

1 onion, chopped

½ teaspoon salt, plus a little extra for cooking the onion

3 cloves garlic, minced

½ teaspoon smoked paprika

1 pound washed and dried collard greens, sliced into ribbons
   (about 1 large bunch)

1 cup vegetable broth

3 cups cooked pinto beans

Pinch of crushed red pepper flakes (or to taste)

Black pepper to taste

For the Tahini Drizzle

¼ cup tahini

¼ cup water

2 tablespoons lemon juice

1 small garlic clove, finely minced

¼ teaspoon salt

Black pepper to taste

- In a large skillet, heat the olive oil over medium heat. Add the onion and a pinch of salt. Sauté, stirring frequently, until the onion is soft, clear, and lightly golden, about 7 to 8 minutes. Add the garlic, paprika, and ½ teaspoon salt. Cook for 2 more minutes.

- Add the collards and broth. Cover the pan and allow the collards to wilt down (you might have to do this in batches). Reduce the heat to medium low, uncover the pan, and cook the collards, stirring every so often, for about 10 minutes. Stir in the pinto beans and a dash of red pepper.

- Season with black pepper to taste.

- To make the tahini drizzle, whisk together all the ingredients.

- Serve the greens and beans in bowls or over cooked brown rice with the tahini drizzle on the side.

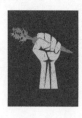

Daily Action 16:

STOCK UP ON VEGAN CONVENIENCE FOODS

Going vegan doesn't mean you have to give up on convenience. There are advantages to cooking foods from scratch, but it's not always an option for everyone. And even for those who have the resources and ability to cook, there are days when we need a little bit of help and some time-saving options. Keep these foods on hand to ensure that you can always pull a healthy meal together no matter the circumstances.

Instant oatmeal
Ready to eat cereals
Plant milks in shelf-stable cartons
Soup cups
Canned beans
Dehydrated refried beans

Precooked microwaveable shelf-stable rice

Frozen precooked rice or other grains

Frozen veggie meats

Vegan macaroni and cheese dinners

Rice-A-Roni and other instant grain mixes (check labels, since not
all are vegan)

Canned or frozen vegetables (including those that are microwaveable in the bag)

Prewashed vegetables in bags

Baked tofu

TVP

Nut butters

Frozen berries

THREE MEALS YOU CAN MAKE
WITH MINIMAL COOKING

- Instant oatmeal with almond milk, walnuts, and frozen berries
  Peanut butter on a bagel

- Tabouli made from a mix with addition of canned chickpeas
  Salad from a bag with bottled dressing

- Rice made with precooked frozen rice
  Refried beans from dehydrated mix or can and topped with salsa
  Cooked frozen spinach

chapter 6

CULTIVATING COMPASSION

In *The Descent of Man*, Charles Darwin suggested that sympathy for others is a stronger instinct than our own self-interest and that this was good for our own evolution as a species. There is evidence that acting in a way that expresses compassion can bolster brain activity in areas associated with feelings of reward. Perhaps that is why compassion feels good, even though the word means "to suffer with." Expressing compassion, we want to help relieve that suffering.

We've all heard someone say, "you can't change the world," as a way to dismiss altruistic concerns and efforts. Believing that you can do something to relieve the suffering of someone else helps you feel more compassionate. Research suggests that compassion grows when you believe you can make a difference. Veganism offers us one place to start, since compassion is at the center of vegan practice for many of us. Through daily tasks of cooking, shopping, and even cleaning, we express compassion by the choices we make. Like a walking meditation, adopting a vegan diet isn't just a way to *express* compassion; it's a way to *build* compassion. You may think that people are either compassionate or they're not. But research suggests that people can grow their compassion. We do this first by looking for what we have in common with someone else and also by seeing others as individuals. Inequality hinders compassion because it's harder to feel compassion when you see yourself as superior to someone else. We also feel less compassion for people when we blame them for their own misfortune.

> **Through daily tasks of cooking, shopping, and even cleaning, we express compassion by the choices we make.**

The 20th-century French mystic Simone Weil wrote: "The love of our neighbor in all its fullness simply means being able to say, 'What are you going through?'" and then being willing to listen to the answer. She writes, "this question is a recognition that the sufferer exists" not as a unit in a collection, or a specimen from the social category labeled "unfortunate," but as an individual who "was one day stamped with a special mark by affliction." To us, this is the basis of compassion.

BANISHMENT OF COMPASSION TO THE PRIVATE WORLD

Over decades, if not centuries, compassion has been banished from the public eye into the private world. In the late 18th century, philosophy turned toward approaches that valued rationalist motivations for behavior and decisions over those that valued "sentiment." As the family evolved during the 19th and 20th centuries, men were encouraged to aim for self-reliance and independence, while systems developed that criticized, mocked, and stereotyped sympathy.

During the last century—especially in that formative decade, the 1950s—caring took on a sentimental aspect and became something for the private sphere not the public. What evolved was a subtle misogyny. Caring was seen as "weak" politically. In *The Way We Never Were*, Stephanie Coontz observes that "Emotion and compassion could be disregarded in the political and economic realms only if women were assigned these traits in the personal realm." As "individualism" and a "survival of the fittest" ethos spread in society, the family became more and more idealized as the site of altruism and love.

As a result, compassion disappeared as an aspect of who we are as politically engaged people. Instead, the assignment of care to the private realm helped to perpetuate, and even reward, a degree of meanness in politics. In the 2016 presidential election in the United States, we saw how willingly people dismissed the importance of compassion, kindness, and sympathy among public figures, and chose to (literally) applaud behavior that most of us would not welcome in our homes.

COMPASSION INCLUDES HOSPITALITY

The dictionary defines *hospitality* as "the friendly reception and treatment of guests or strangers" or "the quality or disposition of receiving and treating guests and strangers in a warm, friendly, generous way." In contrast, *xenophobia*, or "fear of the stranger," perceives only differences, particularly racial and ethnic differences.

Throughout Europe, the question of hospitality has been hotly debated as the European migrant crisis unfolds. Starting in 2011, Syrian refugees began seeking safety from warfare, as did emigrants from Afghanistan and Iraq. In 2015 alone, more than one million migrants and refugees entered European countries, and this migration is expected to continue. Unfortunately, what often greets refugees is not hospitality but panic, fear, and stereotyping as a result of nationalism and xenophobia.

Sociologist Zygmunt Bauman notes that efforts to cast certain groups as unworthy of respect helps to shift focus from the "sphere of ethics to that of threats to security, crime prevention and punishment, criminality, defense of order, and, all in all, the state of emergency usually associated with the threat of military aggression and hostilities." Bauman considers the "moral panic" that politicians appeal to as they stir up xenophobia against refugees and immigrants.

In April 2016 the Southern Poverty Law Center (SPLC), which monitors hate group activity in the United States, surveyed 2,000 teachers across the US about the effect that the presidential elections of that year was having on their students. The teachers reported an increase in anti-immigrant and anti-Muslim comments in their schools. The SPLC called it "The Trump Effect." A follow-up survey after the election, this time of 10,000 teachers, found a dramatic increase in harassment reports since the April survey along with considerable anxiety among minority students.

In both the United States and Europe debates continue about the issue of extending a welcoming hand to strangers or to anyone who isn't "like us." For many, "like us" refers to the ever-shrinking white majority. Freelance writer Jennifer Mendelsohn found a unique way to challenge the anti-immigration stances of U.S. government representatives and others. Her Twitter project #resistancegenealogy reveals the immigrant roots of anti-immigrant politicians. "Unless you're Native American or you descend from slaves who were brought here against their will, you are an immigrant in this country, or you're a descendant of an immigrant in this country," she said.

> ## The ethics of veganism resides in the practice of removing barriers of otherness and viewing all beings with respect.

With compassion at its ethical core, veganism includes a challenge to xenophobia. Within the ethics of veganism resides the practice of removing barriers of otherness and viewing all beings with respect. While a vegan ethic may focus on animals, it can't logically exist without a broader viewpoint that includes all humans and deems everyone worthy of regard. This kind of veganism holds compassion at its center and extends hospitality to all.

COMPASSION FOR ANIMALS

In 1965, novelist Brigid Brophy observed, "Whenever people say, 'We mustn't be sentimental,' you can take it they are about to do something cruel. And if they add, 'We must be realistic,' they mean they are going to make money out of it." While she could easily have been addressing the lack of compassion that is represented by the politics of exclusion, she was talking about animal agriculture.

People are "sentimental" about animals all the time, not just the ones who live with them as pets. Marine rescue units show up to help beached dolphins and whales. People rescue animals in their backyards all the time by calling on wildlife specialists to take injured animals into care and rehabilitate them.

And it's not just wild animals that arouse the desire to help. When a cow escaped a Cincinnati slaughterhouse and ran free for eleven days, eluding animal control authorities, she quickly became a local hero. Upon capture, she went to a sanctuary, not the slaughterhouse. The public concern for animals like her usually comes after media coverage has shone a light on their individuality and desire to live.

Animals on factory farms want to live, too. And they want to be free. But feeling compassion for a group of beings is much harder when they live and die out of our sight. One aspect of the politics of cruelty is that it takes a lot of effort to maintain cruelty and keep it hidden. Animal agriculture enlists politicians to pass laws to keep animal activists out of their operations. Farmers don't want the public to see videos of what goes on behind the walls of their facilities. Or at least they want to restrict those videos to the ones they carefully and selectively create themselves. Sometimes the public is complicit in this. Do we really want to know how animals are treated? Poet and activist Maya Angelou said, "I did then what I knew how to do. Now that I know better, I do better." That's the challenge of knowing about animal agriculture: it presents hard choices, which is why we're often happier not to know.

In his article "Consider the Lobster" in *Gourmet* magazine, David Foster Wallace famously asked, "Is it all right to boil a sentient creature alive just for our gustatory pleasure?" He admits, "The whole animal-cruelty-and-eating issue is not just complex, it's also uncomfortable. It is, at any rate, uncomfortable for me, and for just about everyone I know who enjoys a variety of foods and yet does not want to see herself as cruel and unfeeling. As far as I can tell, my own main way of dealing with these conflicts has been to avoid thinking about the whole unpleasant thing."

Obviously, he's not alone. And in the 21st century, it's likely that most people believe that animal cruelty is rare on farms and there are laws to protect cows, pigs, and chickens. But there aren't. In the United States, animal welfare laws don't protect farmed animals. Most of what happens on a farm—family or factory, organic or conventional—falls outside the criminal code. This includes debeaking chickens without anesthesia, castrating baby pigs without anesthesia, killing male chicks in hatcheries through suffocation or by grinding them alive, and many more practices that are standard procedure on modern farms. If these things were done to a dog or cat, the law would recognize it as animal cruelty. On the farm, it's business as usual and perfectly legal business at that.

The fact that all of these practices are legal makes our responsibility to discern cruelty and to respond to it all the greater.

CONSIDER THE BIRD AND THE FISH

When David Foster Wallace turns his attention from lobsters to farmed animals, he makes a noteworthy observation. "It is significant that 'lobster,' 'fish,' and 'chicken' are our culture's words for both the animal and the meat, whereas most mammals seem to require euphemisms like 'beef' and 'pork' that help us separate the meat we eat from the living creature the meat once was."

There is evidence that people feel a smaller sense of unease—or no sense of unease at all—about eating birds and fishes. This might be one reason why meat-reducers often gravitate away from beef and pork. It feels like a logical place to start. Moving away from these foods is good for health and the environment. It's good for cows and pigs, too. But if you are looking at the issue of how to reduce your meat intake from the perspective of compassion, it's not the logical place to start at all. To make a change that has a significant impact on animal suffering, it makes far better sense to stop eating chickens and fishes.

The Birds

Of the twenty-five animals that the average meat-eater consumes on a yearly basis, twenty-four are birds: chickens and turkeys. Of course, the reason so many chickens are eaten is that they're small. It takes more than 200 chickens to provide the same number of meals as one cow. And, meat from a chicken is popular because of its perceived healthfulness, because it's cheap, and because people like it. The U.S. love affair with chicken meat is such that nearly 130,000 of these animals die for our plates every single hour of the day. Beef intake is on the decline in the United States, but chicken consumption is higher than ever. The result is that while meat intake overall is down, more animals than ever are being killed.

Not only do these animals suffer in huge numbers, but they also suffer mightily.

The Humane Slaughter Act, weak as it is, doesn't even cover birds. That is, they are exempt from laws meant to decrease risk of suffering during death. Although chickens and turkeys are supposed to be dead by the time they are dunked into a scalding bath, because of the speed of slaughterhouse processing lines, they sometimes aren't. According to USDA figures, as many as a million chickens per year may be alive when they are dropped into boiling water.

However, the life of a chicken raised for meat or egg production is dismal even before arriving at the slaughterhouse. They are packed by the tens of thousands into windowless sheds where they live among toxic ammonia fumes from their own filth and may be unable to walk because they are bred to grow so quickly their legs can't support their weight. Dr. John Webster, a former British professor of veterinary science, has described modern chicken production as "the single most severe, systematic example of man's inhumanity to another sentient being," in both its magnitude and severity.

Fishes Feel

Although you may find it difficult to warm up to a fish, science shows that these creatures are more complex than we once realized. Fishes are capable of planning and using tools, and they have long memories. Like only a handful of other animals, including humans, some fishes may be capable of mirror self-recognition. These are sentient creatures who are also capable of suffering.

Fishes for consumption and products from fishes like fish oil supplements may come from fish farms or be captured from the wild. Commercial fishing employs many methods including trawling with nets and use of lines and hooks. Changes in pressure as fishes are rapidly hauled from deep oceans can cause agonizingly painful death. There is no requirement for the humane slaughter of fishes. Most die of asphyxiation in nets or on board ships. Even if you eat a fish's flesh only a couple of times per week, those meals are responsible for the death of many more fishes and other animals than you realize. Hundreds of thousands of sea turtles, seabirds, penguins, and marine mammals, including whales, dolphins, and porpoises, die as bycatch. That is, they are caught along with the target fishes and disposed of. And when you eat farmed fishes, you are also responsible for the death of the more than 100 wild-caught fishes used to feed the one on your plate since it can take hundreds of fishes to feed a single domestically farmed fish.

BULLYING, ANIMALS, AND VEGANISM

Bullying is an expression of power and control. To bully someone, you must first reduce them to an object, to a fragment that you don't need to care about. Bullying arises out of fear, a lack of information, and a culture that objectifies and demeans others, a process that creates barriers to empathy. In 2005, a research study found a connection between bullying and human and animal abuse. The research involved more than 500 children and indicated that schoolyard bullies "were twice as likely to have committed some form of animal abuse when compared to their non-bullying peers." In another study, this one of male college students, those who had been involved in more than one episode of animal abuse were more likely to have been either a victim or a perpetrator of bullying. Those who had been both a victim and a perpetrator were more likely to have been involved in numerous acts of animal abuse and to have a higher tolerance for animal cruelty.

It might seem like a stretch to suggest that animals on factory farms are "bullied." After all, they are there not because we desire to hurt them for the sake of gaining a sense of power, but because we want to eat meat, drink milk, and wear leather. But the environment that allows humans to feel okay about using animals in these ways is starkly similar to the one that invites bullying: We feel a sense of control over the animals and a sense of superiority or entitlement. We reduce them to objects (most animals on farms are identified by a number, not a name) or, as we talked about in chapter 1, to machines.

In order to use animals in ways that we don't require for our own survival, it's necessary to stay uninformed about what they go through on factory farms or, as that becomes increasingly difficult in our information age, to remain desensitized to it. Given what we know about the benefits of compassion for our own species and for individuals, extending that compassion to farmed animals can only be good for all of us.

WHAT WE LEARN FROM ANIMALS' RESISTANCE

Consider this: just as we are resisting regressive politics, the other animals also engage in resistance, with one big difference: their resistance is against us. When they can, they escape from slaughterhouses, dodging humans chasing them as they run down urban streets or hide in forests. A cow who gave birth to twins hid one of her calves so that the farmer would not take the calf away from her to send to a veal farm. She surreptitiously nursed her child for two weeks before the farmer discovered and removed the calf. In New Zealand, lambs unlatch gates and flee. Captive elephants refuse commands even though a bullhook with barbed ends will soon lacerate them. Don't the lobsters who try to crawl out of the pot filled with boiling water try to resist their fate? Pregnant sows placed in gestation crates fight their confinement, sometimes for days.

"Why do you care so much about animal suffering when so many people are suffering?"

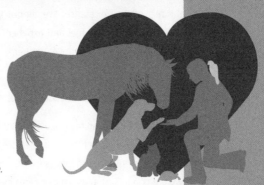

1. Compassion isn't divisible. It's not either/or.

2. Care is about relationships. How we relate to animals doesn't preclude us from relating to humans with compassion.

3. What is happening to animals contributes to human suffering.

4. Animal suffering matters itself as a moral wrong.

5. Some people have excellent skills in helping people; others in caring for animals. We don't ask vets why they aren't brain surgeons. We accept that care for animals is needed.

6. Caring for animals reminds us that suffering is often nonverbal.

7. In caring about animals, we learn of ways to approach rigid hierarchies of human society.

8. Ask yourself, "Who benefits when those struggling for a better world end up fighting with each other?"

9. An assumption hiding behind the question is that people suffering from social oppression don't care about animals. In fact, they do. Homeless individuals have refused shelter if it means abandoning companion animals. Battered women may stay with or return to a violent partner to protect a dog or cat.

WHY WE CARE

An animal's experience of violation matters to that animal. It is the fact of their existence. We cannot know what they know, but we can know what they feel and experience: discomfort, pain, fear, grief, exhaustion, inability to move, hunger.

COMPASSION FOR OURSELVES

Being alert to how animals experience their own lives can cause feelings of overwhelming grief, sadness, and despair. It doesn't have to incapacitate us, though. In some ways it enriches us because it teaches us that we are connected and that our capacity for handling difficult emotions is greater than we might realize.

Jo-Anne McArthur is a photojournalist who has traveled around the world photographing our relationship with animals. Two books of her photographs have been published, *We Animals* and *Captivity*. She has photographed animals in factory farms, slaughterhouses, and family farms and in laboratories, zoos, and circuses. We talked to her about compassion.

When I started seeing, I could not unsee. My job is literally to look these animals in the eye and create a connection with them, so that the audience, the viewer, can also do that through the images. If the animal is looking into the lens, they are looking at the audience. I am trying to gently be there with them and just see a little of their personality, or see a little bit of their anguish and connect with that. And then I have to do it again and again, one animal after the next. The next suffering sow, the next dairy cow who has had her baby taken away, or the next veal calf who doesn't know what is going on because they are just a baby, having been taken from their mothers.

People ask me, "How do you survive it?" I don't always survive. It is inevitable to hurt and suffer from it. I'm scarred. It took a long time to make peace with the fact that I simply go to bear witness and document and that I can't save everyone I meet. For me it has to be enough and that I'm doing my best. That was my process. What I do is educate people. I work really hard to do that and that is my role. I have to be happy in order to do this work, so I focus on the good in people, and on change. I often tell people to nurture and honor their joy because you burn out pretty quickly if you don't.

Being a caring and compassionate person means that we grieve. We grieve for the animals, the environment, for families torn apart by heartless immigration laws, for parents whose children have lost their lives to gun violence, for transgender children who took their own lives because they were bullied. We know, as folksinger and activist Joan Baez says, that "action is the antidote to despair." And so we march, call our representatives, donate to good causes, and volunteer in soup kitchens and animal shelters. We also canvass, plant gardens, vote, and run for office. And we allow ourselves to grieve. But we also learn to develop ways to have compassion for our own grieving selves, celebrate what we are accomplishing, and find ways to nurture joy.

There is always an invitational aspect to caring: an invitation to grow compassion in ourselves and in the world. What if we thought about cultivating compassion as we think about planting a garden? First there is the intention; we identify what is needed, what will we plant? In the case of compassion, it is both the ingredient and the action—so we have to start with the seeds of caring. Gardens need protection, like mulch, nourishment, and water—just as our compassion does: it needs to be tended, which in this case is our own work at enacting compassion. Even when we pull up the roots of tomato plants in the fall, we are still cultivating our garden. Discarding habits that we know now are harmful is akin to the work we do in the fall garden. In this, we make space in our lives to show everyday kindness to those around us and to find both personal and political ways to enact hospitality and compassion to all.

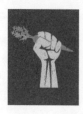

Daily Action 17:

CELEBRATE FOOD OF MIDDLE EASTERN COUNTRIES

Veganism is about compassion, acceptance, inclusiveness, and hospitality. We welcome everyone at our table. Over the past few years, many groups of people have been made to feel far less welcome in the United States. In particular, bigotry against people from Middle Eastern countries has been on the upswing. There is much work to be done to counter that. As we work against Islamophobia and immigrant bashing, we can also celebrate the exceptional food from cultures targeted by anti-immigrant politicians. Here are two of our favorite recipes.

Muhamara

Makes about 2 cups

This traditional Syrian walnut dip is a delicious alternative to hummus. It's worth looking for pomegranate molasses, a condiment that offers a distinctive flavor.

   1 cup roasted red peppers
   1 cup walnuts, lightly toasted
   2 cloves garlic, chopped
   1 teaspoon fresh lemon juice
   ½ teaspoon ground cumin
   1 teaspoon red pepper flakes or to taste
   2 teaspoons pomegranate molasses
   ¼ cup extra-virgin olive oil
   ¼ cup fresh bread crumbs
   Salt to taste
   Pita bread to serve

- Combine the roasted peppers, walnuts, garlic, lemon juice, cumin, red pepper flakes, pomegranate molasses, and olive oil in a food processor. Process until smooth.

- Add the bread crumbs and process just to combine. Season with salt and red pepper flakes to taste.

- Serve with pita bread.

Baba Ganouj

Serves 8 as an appetizer

This popular Middle Eastern dip is usually prepared by charring the eggplant to get a smoky flavor. Our easier version uses a drop or two of liquid smoke.

2 medium eggplants
1 lemon, juiced
¼ cup tahini
3 garlic cloves
¼ cup chopped fresh parsley
1 teaspoon salt
¼ cup green onions, finely minced
1 tablespoon olive oil
Dash of cayenne
1–2 drops liquid smoke
Pita wedges to serve

- Preheat the oven to 400 degrees.

- Wash the eggplants and prick them all over with a fork. Place on a cookie sheet and bake for 45 minutes or until they are soft and wrinkled.

- Let the eggplants cool, and then scoop out the insides. Place in a food processor and add the rest of the ingredients. Process until smooth.

- Chill, and serve with pita wedges.

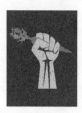

Daily Action 18:

TRY A CHICK'N DISH

Moving meat from chickens and fishes off your plate is one of the most compassionate decisions you can make. Because these animals suffer in such large numbers and are victims of some of the cruelest practices in food production, it's a good place to start.

You can find vegan versions of chicken burgers, chicken nuggets, grilled chicken strips, even buffalo chicken wings—with all the taste and none of the cruelty.

If you want to add chicken-y flavor to your own homemade foods, look for seasonings that were developed specifically for that purpose. Chik-Style Seasoning from Butler Foods or McKay's Vegan Chicken Seasoning are good choices. Dredge tofu cubes or homemade seitan in a mix of flour and one of these seasonings and then fry. No Chicken Base from Better than Bouillon and Not-Chick'n cubes can be used to make broths, sauces, and gravies.

Chicken-Free Potpie

Chicken potpie is a favorite comfort food, and it's easy to create a vegan version. We use sautéed tofu in this recipe, but you can also substitute vegetarian chicken like Gardein Grilled Chicken Strips, or Beyond Meat's Lightly-Seasoned Strips. You can also use chicken-flavored soy curls (see page 65), or you can skip the "meat" altogether and enjoy a vegetable potpie.

8 ounces firm tofu

3 tablespoons vegetable oil, divided

1 tablespoon chicken-flavored seasoning (like Chik-Style Seasoning from Butler Foods or McKay's Vegan Chicken Seasoning),
divided

½ cup diced onion

¼ cup sliced celery

1 carrot, diced

2 cups vegetable broth, divided

1 russet potato, diced

2 cloves garlic, minced

¼ cup all-purpose flour

½ cup fresh or frozen peas

1 teaspoon dried sage

1 teaspoon dried thyme

Salt and pepper

2 premade pie crusts

- Preheat the oven to 400° F.

- Press the tofu between clean kitchen or paper towels to remove as
  much water as possible. Cut into small cubes.

- Heat 1 tablespoon of the olive oil in a large skillet over medium heat
  and cook the tofu until golden, about 10 minutes. Remove the tofu
  from skillet and toss with ½ tablespoon of the chicken-style seasoning mix. Set aside.

- Heat 1 more tablespoon of the oil in the same skillet. Add the onion,
  celery, and carrot, and sauté until the onion is translucent. Add ½
  cup of the vegetable broth, the potato, and the garlic. Cover and
  simmer until the potato is just slightly tender. Remove the vegetables
  from the skillet.

- Heat the remaining tablespoon of oil in the skillet and stir in the
  flour. Cook over medium heat for about two minutes. Slowly pour
  in the remaining vegetable broth, stirring constantly to keep lumps

from forming. Stir in the remaining chicken-style seasoning. Cook over medium heat until the sauce starts to thicken. Add the tofu, vegetables, peas, sage, and thyme and stir to coat with the gravy.

- Season with the salt and pepper.

- Pour the mixture into one of the pie crusts. With a rolling pin or your hands, flatten the second pie crust and place it on top of the vegetables. Crimp the edges. Cut an X in the middle of the top crust.

- Bake until crust is golden and the gravy is bubbling, about 30 minutes.

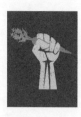

Daily Action 19:
TRY A VEGAN FISH DISH

Dried sea vegetables (more commonly called seaweeds) offer a simple and effective way to create a "fishlike" flavor in recipes. Sea vegetables are packed with nutrients and flavor and are a sustainable type of seafood. For this vegan tuna salad recipe, we used Kelp Granules from the Maine Coast Sea Vegetables company.

NoTuna Salad

Serves 4

This fast chickpea spread is perfect for sandwiches or served on a bed of lettuce for a light lunch.

1½ cups cooked chickpeas (or one 15-ounce can, drained and rinsed)
¼ cup chopped celery
¼ cup finely chopped onion
1 tablespoon fresh lemon juice
¼ cup vegan mayonnaise

½ tablespoon kelp granules

2 tablespoons chopped fresh parsley (optional)

Salt and pepper to taste

Whole-grain bread to serve

Sliced tomato to serve

- Process the chickpeas in a food processor, or mash with a potato masher, until coarsely chopped. Transfer to a bowl.

- Stir in the rest of the ingredients. Adjust the seasonings as needed. Serve on whole-grain bread with sliced tomatoes.

Daily Action 20:

BRING CHILDREN TO AN ANIMAL SANCTUARY (OR BRING A SANCTUARY TO THEM)

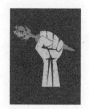

Children have a natural affinity for animals. Instead of taking them to a petting zoo—an encounter that teaches that their experience is more important than the animals' experience of captivity—give them an opportunity to see animals in settings that honor their inherent dignity. Farm animal sanctuaries are able to save only a small number of animals from today's factory farms. But their essential work allows people to connect with individual cows, goats, pigs, turkeys, and chickens, giving visitors the opportunity to learn more about why the work to liberate animals from factory farms is so important. You can find a list of these sanctuaries at *www.vegan.com/farm-sanctuaries*.

In addition to farm sanctuaries, there are safe havens for wild animals. If you can't get to one of these places in person, there are ways to bring the experience right into your home. Visit the lions and bears of the Wild Animal Sanctuary in Colorado through their video series at *www.wildanimalsanctuary.org*, or help schoolchildren take a virtual field trip to the Elephant Sanctuary in Tennessee through their distance learning program on *www.elephantsanctuary.org*.

Chocolate Chip Cookies

Makes 18 cookies

Nothing goes together quite like kids and cookies and a field trip! Whether at home or on the road, these are wonderful cookies to bring along.

The secret to making the best chocolate chip cookies is to let the dough rest overnight before baking. Make these to pack up for a car trip to an animal sanctuary.

2 cups all-purpose flour

1 teaspoon baking powder

¾ teaspoon baking soda

½ teaspoon fine salt

1¼ cups vegan chocolate chips

½ cup organic sugar

½ cup packed light or dark brown sugar

½ cup plus 1 tablespoon canola, grapeseed, or any other neutral oil

¼ cup plus 1 tablespoon water

Coarse-grained sea salt for garnish

- In a large bowl, whisk together the flour, baking powder, baking soda, and salt. Add the chocolate chips to the flour mixture and toss to coat.

- In a separate large bowl, whisk the sugars briskly with the canola oil and water until smooth and incorporated, about 2 minutes.

- Add the flour mixture to the sugar mixture, and then stir with a wooden spoon or a rubber spatula until just combined and no flour is visible. Do not overmix.

- Cover with plastic wrap. Refrigerate the dough for at least 12 hours and up to 24 hours. Do not skip this step.

- Preheat the oven to 350° F. Line two rimmed baking sheets with parchment paper. Remove the dough from the refrigerator and use an ice-cream scoop or a spoon to portion it into 2-inch mounds. We recommend freezing the balls of dough for 10 minutes before baking as the cookies will retain their shape better that way.

- Sprinkle the balls of dough with coarse-grained sea salt (after you remove balls of dough from the freezer if you took this step), and bake for 12 to 13 minutes, or until the edges are just golden. Do not overbake.

- Let the cookies cool completely before serving.

Daily Action 21:
CHOOSE AN ACTIVITY THAT CONNECTS YOU WITH ANIMALS IN NEED

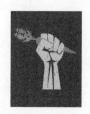

There are so many ways to help animals, including activities for those who are short on time.

- Attend a slaughterhouse vigil or a circus protest.

- Gather food and bedding to donate to a shelter or a wildlife rescue and rehab.

- Sign up with a local Community Cats program to feed colonies of feral cats.

- Put up a bird feeder.

- Put out a heated water bowl for wildlife during winter freezes.

Peanut Butter Dog Biscuits (for the World-wide Vegan Bake Sale)

Yield will vary based on size of your cookie cutter.

Between April 15 and 30 (or at any time!) groups and individuals around the world hold Vegan Bake Sales to support their favorite causes. Since 2009, people have raised more than $360,000 to donate to nonprofit organizations. Anyone can participate. Just choose a venue, decide what you want to sell, and choose who you want to donate the money to. Many people donate to local animal shelters. One fun way to raise money is to sell homemade vegan dog biscuits.

> 2 cups whole-wheat flour
> ½ cup cornmeal
> ½ cup oats
> ½ cup oil
> 3 tablespoons peanut butter
> 2 teaspoons vanilla extract
> 1½ cups water

- Preheat the oven to 400 degrees.

- In a large bowl, combine the flour, cornmeal, and oats. Stir in the oil, peanut butter, vanilla, and water. Knead until smooth, adding more flour and water as needed.

- Roll onto a lightly floured surface and cut with cookie cutters. Bake on a greased cookie sheet for 20 minutes.

Homemade Vegan Birdseed Blocks

Makes 24 small blocks

Birdseed blocks are usually made with suet, a product of factory farming. It's easy to make your own with ice cube trays and a fun project for kids. They also make great gifts!

1½ cups vegetable shortening or coconut oil
¾ cups nut butter (any kind)
3½ cups wild birdseed
1 cup quick oats
½ cup cornmeal

- Combine the shortening and nut butter in a pan and melt over low heat.

- Mix together the birdseed, oats, and cornmeal.

- Pour the melted mixture over the seed mixture and stir to combine. Spoon into ice cube trays and freeze for two hours. Place the cubes in a suet feeder to feed the birds.

chapter 7

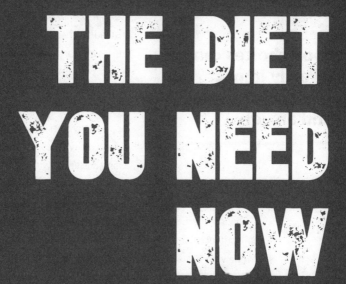

THE DIET
YOU NEED
NOW

THE ANTISTRESS AND ANTIDEPRESSION DIET YOU NEED NOW

"How do you stay outraged without losing your mind?" asked feminist attorney Mirah Curzer in a blog post shortly after the 2016 election. It's also a question that vegans have been asking for decades. Burnout, depression, compassion fatigue, and information overload are issues that are all too familiar to activists. Veganism is a response to information about the lives of animals in agriculture, research, and entertainment. The sheer volume of suffering is overwhelming. How do you stay focused and determined without becoming overwhelmed and stressed? How do you avoid burnout? How do you stay abreast of the news but still manage to ward off the blues when the news is so depressing?

One way is to periodically detach and disengage from the news. We have learned that we don't have to know about every single bad thing happening to animals in order to work against those things. It's the same with the political news. You might turn off your CNN and *New York Times* news alerts, choosing instead to check the news once per day. You might focus on just one or two issues and choose to be less informed about the others. Getting your news from newspapers rather than television gives you the opportunity to skim and pick and choose what you want to consume rather than being presented with a buffet of information and discussion that you might not want to hear. You also might take a complete break from the news for several days each week.

Food choices can directly impact feelings of depression and anxiety.

That's just a first step, though. It's also essential for you, as part of the resistance, to bring some focus to your self-care. It's essential for anyone who has a busy and demanding life, in fact. Getting adequate sleep, choosing restorative exercise like yoga or walking, and embracing activities like meditation, prayer, journaling or talking to a friend or mental health professional can ease stress. Time spent on these pursuits is time well spent since self-care is crucial if you want to be effective in your other activities.

Eating well is a critical part of an effective self-care routine. While little indulgences can bring an immediate sense of much-needed comfort, you know that a steady diet of junk foods makes you feel sluggish and tired. There is also a growing body of evidence to suggest that food choices can directly impact feelings of depression and anxiety. Nutrition researchers have found that people eating traditional plant-based diets, like healthy Mediterranean and Japanese-style diets, are at lower risk for depression. Those eating vegetarian diets may have lower risk also. The evidence points to the protective effects of plant foods that sit at the center of these eating patterns—fruits, vegetables, beans, nuts and seeds, healthy fats, tea and red wine, and fiber-rich foods.

DIET AND INFLAMMATION

Stress and depression are both linked to systemic inflammation. Unlike the redness and swelling that occur around an injury like a swollen ankle, you can't feel this type of inflammation, but it's believed to be an underlying factor in heart disease, diabetes, cancer, and Alzheimer's disease.

Its relationship to depression, stress, and anxiety seems to be a two-way street, though. Being depressed or chronically anxious can raise levels of inflammation, which may be one reason why depression raises the risk for heart disease and diabetes. But inflammation may also be an underlying cause of depression or at least it may make depression worse. Many of the lifestyle habits that are effective in reducing symptoms of depression and anxiety, like meditation and exercise, happen to also reduce inflammation.

This leads us to believe that a diet that reduces inflammation could also reduce some types of depression. And there is evidence to suggest that this is true.

PLANT FOODS AND ANTIOXIDANTS

As cells burn glucose for energy, they produce damaging oxygen-containing compounds called free radicals. Free radicals attack cells and impair their function, setting off a chain reaction that leads to a condition called oxidative stress. Oxidative stress in turn promotes inflammation.

You can't stop free radical production since it's a consequence of normal metabolism. But you can interfere with the damage it does to cells. In particular, plant foods are packed with the antioxidant compounds that neutralize these free radicals. For example, the beta-carotene that gives carrots and sweet potatoes their bright orange color is a powerful antioxidant. Since it also gets turned into vitamin A in the body, this compound does double duty for your health, as both a vitamin and an antioxidant. In contrast, the vitamin A in animal foods doesn't show any antioxidant activity.

> **Replacing meat, dairy, and eggs in your diet is almost guaranteed to boost your antioxidant intake, and this may have real impact on the risk of depression.**

Brightly colored fruits and vegetables—leafy greens, red cabbage, winter squash, and berries—are especially rich in antioxidants, but all whole plant foods including nuts, seeds, whole grains, and beans have them. Replacing meat, dairy, and eggs in your diet is almost guaranteed to boost your antioxidant intake, and this may have real impact on the risk of depression.

CARBS AND FATS AND INFLAMMATION

The kind of fat you eat can impact inflammation, too. Red meat in particular is a source of a fat called arachidonic acid that produces pro-inflammation compounds. Technically, the fat found in most vegetable oils can be converted into arachidonic acid, but the amount of arachidonic acid in your bloodstream is related more strongly to the amount of meat you eat, not how much plant fat you eat.

One plant fat may be especially valuable and that's olive oil. The compound in good-quality extra-virgin olive oil that creates that peppery feeling at the back of your throat is called oleocanthal. It's a phytochemical that reduces inflammation.

Carbohydrates can affect inflammation, too. Carbohydrates enter your bloodstream as glucose, which is sometimes referred to as blood sugar. Glucose is a critical source of fuel for your brain and central nervous system, and your body absolutely needs it. But excessive levels of glucose also promote oxidative stress and inflammation. The way to avoid spikes in glucose levels is not to avoid all carbs; it's to emphasize slowly digested carbs. Plant foods that are minimally processed and rich in fiber release glucose more gradually and produce a gentle, slow rise in blood glucose. While eating too many refined carbohydrates raises risk for depression, eating whole, fiber-rich plant foods lowers it.

All of these factors—eating lots of fruits and vegetables and choosing good-quality plant fats and slow carbs while cutting back on meat—can lead to lower levels of inflammation in your body.

THE SEROTONIN CONNECTION

Serotonin is a neurotransmitter, a compound that carries signals between nerves. Boosting serotonin can improve mood while low levels of this compound may be linked to depression. The most common class of drugs used to treat depression helps maintain serotonin levels.

The extent to which these drugs improve mental health is debated and, in fact, so is the relationship of serotonin to depression. But while we wait for the research to evolve, there are simple dietary choices you can make to ensure that your body has what it needs to make serotonin.

Serotonin is made from the amino acid tryptophan. That's why warm milk, which is rich in tryptophan and perceived by many as a soothing drink, is a popular bedtime snack. There is more to the story than a good supply of tryptophan, though. This amino acid can't get into the brain unless it's escorted by carbohydrates. Carb-rich foods that also provide plenty of tryptophan are the best bet for maintaining serotonin production. Foods that are rich in both tryptophan and carbohydrates include beans, oats, and potatoes. You might be better off with a warm cup of oatmeal than a glass of milk at bedtime.

Building up serotonin levels is one approach to managing stress, anxiety, and depression. Another is to slow the rate at which this neurotransmitter is broken down. A compound in plant foods called quercetin can inhibit the enzyme responsible for degrading serotonin. Foods that are especially high in quercetin are citrus fruits, apples, onions, parsley, tea, red wine, olive oil, grapes, cherries, blueberries, and blackberries. This might be one reason why in a study titled "Many Apples a Day Keep the Blues Away," young adults reported feeling happiest on the days after they ate plenty of fruits and vegetables.

Just how much you can protect your serotonin levels by eating beans and berries isn't known at this point. But there's no doubt that these foods are good for you. If they end up protecting your mood, that's just a bonus.

TOFU AND DEPRESSION

A number of studies show that estrogen therapy can alleviate depression in women after menopause. This has raised questions about compounds in soybeans called isoflavones.

We talked about soy isoflavones in chapters 2 and 4. They are plant estrogens, and while they are close cousins to the female hormone, they aren't exactly the same. But given their likeness to estrogen, it's logical to ask if they might have beneficial effects on depression. There is evidence that the answer is yes. When a group of women consumed isoflavone supplements for ten weeks, their moods improved. The improvements were similar to women taking antidepressants. Taking antidepressant medication plus isoflavones was even better. Studies in Italy and Japan showed similar benefits. In the Japanese study, a daily dose of isoflavones that is about the same as the amount found in one cup of soy milk or a half cup of tofu was enough to have an effect.

We don't know if soyfoods would have the same benefits in men; so far, that hasn't been tested. But again, it's worth a try, especially since soyfoods are linked to lower risk for prostate cancer.

SUPPLEMENTS TO RELIEVE SADNESS

Three nutrients, vitamin B12, vitamin D, and omega-3 fats, may be linked to depression.

If you don't spend much time outdoors during the daylight hours or if you (wisely) use sunscreen, you may not make enough vitamin D. In that case, taking a supplement could help ward off depression since people with low blood levels of vitamin D are more likely to be depressed.

A deficiency of vitamin B12 can result in neurological problems, including depression. When you're cutting back on animal foods for any reason, you may not get enough vitamin B12 since it doesn't occur naturally in plants. In addition, everyone over the age of 50, regular meat-eaters or not, is advised to supplement with B12.

Finally, omega-3 fats may reduce symptoms of depression. These are the fatty acids found in certain cold-water fish and in fish oil supplements, and also in vegan supplements made from algae. (We talk more in the next chapter about vitamin B12, vitamin D, and omega-3 fats, and the steps you can take to make sure you're getting enough.)

EATING TO IMPROVE MOOD: DOES IT REALLY WORK?

As we dig through all of these dietary relationships, a clear picture starts to emerge of how you can eat to protect mood. These are the components of a healthy diet aimed at reducing stress and depression:

- Eat plenty of fruits and vegetables, especially brightly colored ones. Be sure to include a serving or two of fruits or vegetables that are rich in quercetin, the phytochemical that may interfere with breakdown of serotonin. Good choices are oranges, grapefruit, apples, onions, grapes, and berries.

- Choose good-quality, extra-virgin olive oil in place of fats from animal foods.

- Eat beans and potatoes. They provide the amino acid tryptophan plus carbs, necessary for making serotonin and getting it into your brain.

- Have a serving or two of soyfoods every day.

- Protect your brain with supplements: vitamin D, vitamin B12, and algae-derived omega-3 fats.

Eating lots of salads with olive oil dressing, taking a few supplements, and enjoying baked tofu are not enough to counteract all of the stresses of life or cure depression in everyone. Mental health is much more complex than that. You need exercise, adequate sleep, and social engagement to buoy your mood. And some of us will also need medication and/or professional therapy. But the dietary approach to good mental health consists of easy, healthy changes—things that everyone should be doing anyway. And the evidence tells us that they really may help.

PLANT-BASED DIETS, CLIMATE CHANGE, AND HEALTH

Air pollution seems to be associated with either depression or mood, most likely because it contributes to oxidative stress. In contrast, nature provides us with natural substances that may help alleviate stress and depression. Japanese researchers suggest that we are taking in these beneficial substances, including beneficial bacteria and plant-derived essential oils, when we breathe the air in pollution-free surroundings.

The World Health Organization agrees. In their report "Connecting Global Priorities—Biodiversity and Human Health," they said that climate change affects biodiversity in ways that may impact human health, including mental health. We've already seen in chapter 2 that eating more plant foods in place of animal products is a way to reduce global warming and protect biodiversity. It's one more way that your food choices might ease depression.

PEACE OF MIND

"Now I can at last look at you in peace. I don't eat you anymore." These were the words of early 20th-century writer Franz Kafka, while viewing fish in an aquarium. He had recently adopted a vegetarian diet.

Many people, when they stop eating and using animals, report that they feel a sense of deep personal peace. Adopting a vegan diet brings your choices and actions in line with those same beliefs that underlie a commitment to resisting regressive politics: generosity, compassion, and a commitment to justice and fairness. By acting in a way that reflects your values and what you believe, you relieve the cognitive dissonance that can make stress and depression worse. We have a sense of how important it is for people to act in ways that align with their beliefs from studies on death and dying. When people who are dying talk about their biggest regrets, a common one is this: "I wish I'd had the courage to live a life true to myself."

> **By acting in a way that reflects your values and what you believe, you relieve the cognitive dissonance that can make stress and depression worse.**

It's remarkable to see the ways in which such a simple decision—to replace animal foods with plant foods—impacts mental well-being. The plant foods in your diet may have a direct influence on mood. Choosing these foods also contributes to a global environment that may be better for mental health. And a shift in diet brings your habits in closer alliance

Real-Life Tips from Vegans

We asked vegans on social media what they do to stay happy, balanced, and steady as they work to resist regressive politics. Their answers were fun and sometimes funny, inspiring, and hopeful. We share some of their responses here:

- *Laugh. About everything possible. And love those near me.*

- *Walk, cook, and clean.*

- *Make art.*

- *Read mystery books.*

- *Love more, try to learn as much as I can, and spend time every day doing a bit to change things for all of us animals. I also remind myself that the pendulum doesn't swing in only one direction.*

- *Learn to play the ukulele.*

- *Try to focus on the positive actions people take, meet up with like-minded people, read, connect with nature, switch off.*

- *Rescue kittens.*

- *Stay extra close with my dogs, knit, read books on meditation.*

- *Become a Presbyterian.*

- *Hike, bird-watch, give, act.*

- *Try to do something kind for someone every day.*

- *Volunteer for organizations that provide food to poor people.*

- *Notice the skies, trees, mountains, and other elements of nature.*

- *Study history to better understand what we are up against.*

- *Read poetry.*

- *Exercise.*

with your beliefs, which in itself produces a feeling of peace. No matter how you look at it, a vegan diet has extraordinary consequences for your own well-being.

SELF-CARE FOR RESISTING STRESS AND DEPRESSION

Those of us who are willing to do the difficult work of challenging misogyny, bigotry, environmental destruction, animal cruelty, and bullying are in this for the long haul. The work of justice and resistance is hard, and it often seems to advance much too slowly. If we want to be effective and successful, we need to be strong and resilient, and that requires self-care.

Make time to connect with the things that enrich your life—reading, hobbies, sharing with friends and family. Do what it takes to let go of stress and anxiety. In addition to making time for the things you enjoy and letting go of the news you don't enjoy, there are tried-and-true methods for tamping down anxiety and stress. Meditation and breathing exercises, prayer, writing in a journal, and walking outside are simple approaches to stress management that really do work. You don't have to do them all; just find what works for you and then make it a habit.

> **Adopting a vegan diet brings your choices and actions in line with those same beliefs that underlie a commitment to resisting regressive politics.**

WHEN YOU CAN'T DO IT ALL

We resisters want to do whatever we can to turn the tide: we are still protesting, still calling our representatives, still scraping together money to send to organizations, still working with local and national groups to make changes in our communities and beyond. And now, in this book we're calling on change-makers to recognize the impact of altering your diet to help create a more just world. We cannot do it all. Even knowing that, we feel guilty for not doing enough.

One of the best things about a vegan diet is that it means you are doing something at least three times a day that is a part of the resistance and contributes to a world that is just, fair, and kind to animals, the earth, and other people. On the days when you can't fit in one more task beyond work, errands, and family obligations, choosing a hummus wrap for lunch instead of a tuna sandwich is enough. Pouring almond milk over your morning cereal instead of cow's milk is enough. Buying a package of veggie burgers instead of a pound of ground beef at the grocery store is enough.

When you recognize how impactful these choices are and how much you are already doing, it allows you to make room for the things that nourish your soul and maintain some balance in your life. Time to connect with loved ones, to create, or to simply sit back and do nothing is essential for most of us to replenish our mental resources, just like a healthy diet replenishes our physical needs. You need to do it to stay strong for the resistance.

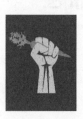

Daily Action 22:

MANAGE YOUR DIET OF NEWS

If you're a news junkie, try an experiment to see if less news will translate to more happiness for you. Turn off TV and internet alerts. Consider downloading a program like Freedom that turns off your internet connection for whatever period of time you determine. Unfollow or mute friends on social media who share fake news or information that isn't useful or productive. Limit your access to information that is useful and less stressful.

This doesn't mean you have to tune out completely. Again, this is where we can learn from vegans. Animal activists want to stay informed because it allows us to adjust our personal consumption choices and also speak out on behalf of animals. We can do that without scrolling through social media feeds filled with distressing photos of abused animals. We follow other activists and organizations we trust to share truthful, helpful information—knowing that sometimes the information is distressing—but tune out the more relentless purveyors of bad news about animals. You can do the same with political news. Identify a few trusted sources and check in with them once or twice a day.

Daily Action 23:
TAKE A HIKE

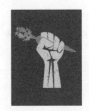

We all know the importance of moving our bodies. Exercise of any type is associated with improved mood. But it's even better if you can get outside. Walking on the beach, in the mountains, a city park, or your backyard creates a feeling of well-being. The Japanese call this *shinrin-yoku* which translates roughly to "forest bathing." It might just be the view or the fact that you are away from the normal pressures and stress of work and home. It might be those beneficial bacteria or the scent of fresh pine or cut grass. It may be beneficial, as well, if you can get away from urban areas and pollution. Even a few minutes outdoors can boost your mood.

Daily Action 24:
MAKE THE SWITCH FROM BUTTER TO EXTRA-VIRGIN OLIVE OIL

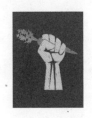

This is a small change that will reduce your intake of saturated fat (at least by a little) and help you take a small but significant step away from animal foods. Good-quality olive oil lies at the heart of Mediterranean cooking. It most likely contributes to the renowned health benefits of this eating style, and it definitely contributes to the culinary appeal of these dishes. Olive oil is associated with a reduced risk for heart disease and possibly some types of cancer.

The key here is "good-quality" olive oil. Make sure the olive oil is labeled "extra-virgin" and look for bottles that show the date of harvest (not to be confused with a "best by" date). Olive oil does not improve with time, so try to buy oil with a harvest date within the past year. It should be in a dark bottle and needs to be stored away from light and heat. Keep in mind that the anti-inflammation compound oleocanthal in olive oil has a bitter or peppery bite to it and you should be able to taste that. If you're lucky enough to have an olive oil boutique nearby that allows tastings, it's a fun and foolproof way to purchase olive oil. Otherwise, we recommend consulting the list of good-quality supermarket olive oils on the Extra Virginity website.

You already know that olive oil makes the best salad dressings and is ideal for sautéing onions or mushrooms. Here are some other ways to switch out butter for olive oil.

- Invest in a good oil spray bottle and use it to spray olive oil on bread instead of spreading butter.

- Infuse olive oil with dried herbs and dip your bread in it Mediterranean style.

- Substitute olive oil in baked goods that call for melted butter or other liquid oils. If the recipe calls for melted butter, substitute with olive oil but use just 75 percent of the amount called for. For example, if the recipe calls for 8 tablespoons of melted butter, use 6 tablespoons of olive oil. You may be surprised to discover how much depth and flavor a robust olive oil can contribute to chocolate desserts.

Orange Almond Olive Oil Cake

Serves 12

A version of this cake, which brings together fresh Mediterranean flavors of citrus, almonds, and olive oil, is found in the cookbook *Vegan Chocolate* by Fran Costigan.

⅓ cup extra-virgin olive oil, plus oil for pan

¾ cup organic unbleached all-purpose flour

½ cup organic whole-wheat pastry flour

¾ cup organic sugar, grind if coarse

1 teaspoon baking soda

½ teaspoon fine sea salt

¼ teaspoon aluminum-free baking powder

⅓ cup very finely ground whole toasted almonds, plus 3 tablespoons

1 cup fresh orange juice

2 tablespoon finely grated orange zest

1 tablespoon apple cider vinegar

½ teaspoon pure vanilla extract

½ teaspoon pure almond extract

2–3 tablespoons coarsely chopped almonds for garnish

- Preheat the oven to 350 degrees. Oil an 8-inch springform pan and line the bottom with parchment cut to fit. Do not oil the parchment.

- Sift together the flours, sugar, baking soda, salt, and baking powder. Add ⅓ cup of the ground almonds and stir with a wire whisk to distribute the ingredients.

- In a separate bowl, combine the orange juice, oil, zest, vinegar, and vanilla and almond extracts, and whisk until well combined. Pour this into the dry mixture and whisk until the batter is smooth.

- Pour the batter into the prepared pan. Rotate the pan to level the batter and tap it lightly on the counter. Bake 35 to 40 minutes, or until the top of the cake is uniformly golden brown, the sides have pulled away from the pan, and a tester inserted in the center of the cake is clean. The cake will compact while cooling.

- Place the cake pan on a cooling rack. Run a thin knife between the cake and pan. Cool 5 minutes and release the side ring. Sprinkle a tablespoon of ground almonds on the cake. Place the cooling rack on top of the cake and invert. Remove the pan and paper. Expect the bottom to be pale and moist. Sprinkle with 1–2 tablespoons of the ground almonds and cool completely.

Oven-Roasted Tomatoes

The sun-dried tomatoes you buy in the store are often packaged in low-quality oil. It's easy to make your own, and while it's a long process—something to do on a lazy Sunday afternoon, perhaps—the actual hands-on preparation is only about 10 minutes. And your kitchen will smell like heaven.

20 Roma tomatoes
2 tablespoons extra-virgin olive oil
2 tablespoons balsamic vinegar
1 to 2 teaspoons dried Italian herb mix
1 to 2 teaspoons sugar (amount depends on how sweet your
    tomatoes are)

- Preheat the oven to 250 degrees.
- Cut the tomatoes in half lengthwise and place cut-side up on a cookie sheet. Sprinkle with remaining ingredients. Bake until the tomatoes are slightly shriveled but still somewhat juicy, about 6 hours.

Daily Action 25:
CHOOSE "SLOW CARBS"

If you suffer from carbophobia, this is a healthy way to invite these foods back into your life. If you're a carb-lover, it's a way to make better choices. There is a world of difference between refined carbs and the ones that come from whole plant foods.

Refined carbohydrates, like sugars, white rice, and foods made from refined flours, can result in elevated blood glucose levels, which can lead to oxidative stress and inflammation. But the carbs in beans, sweet potatoes, and many whole grains don't have that effect, and because they are rich in fiber, it's important to include them in your diet.

The key is to choose carbohydrate-rich foods that are digested slowly so that they result in a more gradual, healthy rise in blood glucose. Generally speaking, this means cutting back on refined, processed carbs and eating more whole plant foods. But even among whole plant foods, some choices are better than others.

SLOW CARBS

Choose these foods	More often than these
Whole grains	Refined grains
Beans cooked from scratch	Canned beans
Bread made from whole, cracked, or sprouted grains	Bread made from flour
Baked potatoes in skin	Mashed potatoes
Whole raw fruits	Cooked or dried fruits or juice
Spaghetti, oats, barley	Rice
Foods flavored with acidic ingredients like lemon, lime, vinegar, or tomatoes	Foods flavored with sweet sauces

Quinoa Confetti Salad

Serves 4 as a main dish salad

This salad is packed with protein from the quinoa and beans and gets plenty of pleasant crunch and color from the raw vegetables.

2 cups water

1 cup quinoa

½ cup diced red onion

1 red bell pepper

1 green bell pepper

1 carrot

1 fresh or canned jalapeño pepper, seeded and minced

2 cups fresh or defrosted frozen corn

¼ cup extra-virgin olive oil

2 tablespoons fresh lemon or lime juice

Salt and fresh ground pepper to taste

1½ cups cooked or canned small red beans

¼ cup chopped fresh parsley

- Bring the water to a boil and add quinoa. Reduce the heat, cover, and simmer until the water is absorbed and the quinoa is tender, about 20 minutes. (If you have a rice maker, you can prepare the quinoa in it; the setting should be "white rice.")

- While the quinoa is cooking, coarsely chop the bell peppers and carrot. Combine the chopped vegetables with the diced onions and minced jalapeños with the corn in a large bowl. Add the oil, lemon juice, salt, and pepper and combine thoroughly.

- Add the cooked quinoa and the beans and toss to combine. Stir in the parsley. Serve warm.

Daily Action 26:

CREATE A COMFORT DRINK

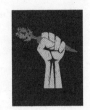

Sitting quietly for a few minutes and sipping a hot soothing drink can go a long way in melting away stress, especially when you're feeling busy and overextended. A plain cup of tea or coffee can sometimes do the trick; both are packed with stress-reducing antioxidants. But for a change of pace, try one of our favorites below.

Ginger Lemon Tea

3 cups water
2-inch piece of fresh gingerroot, peeled and sliced
¼ cup fresh lemon juice
Optional sweetener of your choice

- Combine the water and ginger in a pan and bring to a boil. Remove from heat.

- Add the lemon juice, cover, and let steep for at least 20 minutes. The longer it steeps, the more pronounced the ginger flavor will be. Gently reheat before serving.

Green Matcha Tea Latte with Vanilla and Lavender Syrup

Makes 1 serving

Matcha is a type of green tea that is especially high in antioxidants and caffeine. Carol was introduced to this drink at a small coffee shop in Humboldt, California. She was hooked! Carol likes the vanilla syrup from Williams-Sonoma and the lavender syrup made by L'Épicerie de Provence. This has become the most popular drink in her household.

1 teaspoon matcha

¼ cup hot water (not boiling)

1 cup hot, but not boiling unsweetened plant milk (combine different varieties for fun)

1 tablespoon vanilla syrup

1 tablespoon lavender syrup

- Place the tea in a small bowl. Whisk in the hot water until the tea is dissolved.

- Pour the hot milk into a cup (or heat the milk in the cup in a microwave).

- Add the matcha, lavender, and vanilla syrup to the hot milk. If you have a handheld frother, use that to mix the ingredients and create a froth, or whisk them together.

Healthy Hot Chocolate

Makes 2 servings

Carol's nephew, Jake Fry, introduced her to this quick and tasty alternative to hot chocolate. If you are using a high-speed blender, you don't need to soak the cashews. If using a regular blender, soak the cashews overnight before making this.

½ cup raw cashews (soaked overnight if using a regular blender)

2 cups boiling water

2 dates

2 tablespoons cacao nibs

1 tablespoon lavender syrup (optional)

Combine all of the ingredients in a blender and blend at high speed until completely mixed.

chapter 8

FEEDING YOUR RESISTANCE

If you spend any time browsing vegan topics on the internet, it's easy to be convinced that veganism is a weight loss diet—or maybe a way to make yourself "bulletproof" against disease. It's certainly true that shifting toward more plant-based choices can improve your health. But the benefits of moving toward veganism go so much deeper than that and are so remarkably unique. There are other diets that will help you to lose weight or lower your cholesterol, but none that allow you to make the kind of meaningful choices we've talked about in this book— choices that reflect values about your relationship to other people, other animals, and the earth.

How far you wish to go is up to you. Every time you replace an animal food with a plant-based choice, you have an impact. In this chapter, we'll summarize and expand on some of the earlier daily actions to give you tools to "veganize" just about any recipe. We also provide tips for eating away from home and for setting yourself up for success regarding dietary changes. But first, knowing that your nutrient needs are covered is essential to gaining the confidence to forge ahead.

VEGAN NUTRITION

Protein from Plants

Protein is abundant in the plant world. Certain foods like soyfoods and beans are packed with it, and even grains and vegetables provide respectable amounts of this nutrient.

Our protein requirement is actually for the amino acids that serve as building blocks of protein. Some of these amino acids, referred to as "essential," must come from food since we can't make them ourselves. All plant foods—all grains, vegetables, nuts, seeds, and beans—provide all of the essential amino acids. Even fruits provide them—although not in especially significant quantities.

Nutrition experts once thought that we needed to eat plant foods in certain combinations—like beans with grains—to get the right pattern of amino acids. More recent discoveries show that this isn't true. You'll still see articles about protein combining or protein complementing on the internet, but it's an outdated concept.

Assuming you are getting enough calories, the only rule for meeting protein needs on a vegan diet is to make sure that you eat at least two to three servings per day of legumes. These foods include cooked dried beans and lentils; soyfoods like soy milk, tofu, TVP, and tempeh; and peanuts and peanut butter. If you've been attempting the daily actions in this book, then beans and soyfoods already feel more familiar. Eating three servings of legumes is as simple as having peanut butter on a bagel for breakfast, a hummus wrap for lunch, and a veggie burger for dinner.

The following chart shows serving sizes for the three types of legumes.

Legumes	
Dried beans	½ cup of black beans, navy beans, pinto beans, lima beans, kidney beans, chickpeas, great northern beans, cranberry beans, lentils, split peas
Soyfoods	½ cup of tofu, TVP, tempeh, or edamame or 1 cup soy milk or ¼ cup dried soy nuts
Peanuts	¼ cup shelled peanuts or 2 tablespoons of peanut butter or ¼ cup peanut powder

Healthy Bones: Calcium and Vitamin D (and Protein and Fruits and Vegetables)

With both financial and promotional help from the U.S. Department of Agriculture, the dairy industry has managed to convince us that milk is a dietary essential. It's true that you need calcium—which milk provides—for strong bones. But milk, cheese, and yogurt are not the only foods that provide this nutrient.

A number of plant foods are good sources of calcium, but the amount of calcium in a food is only part of the story. How much of that calcium you absorb matters, too. In fact, if you start looking at the wide variation in calcium content in different foods and the wide variation in absorption rates, it quickly becomes overwhelming. Fortunately, you don't need to pay attention to those details. Instead, just make sure you aim to consume two cups—three if you're over fifty—per day of foods that provide well-absorbed calcium. These include fortified plant milks, fortified fruit juices, tofu made with a calcium salt (look for the words *calcium sulfate* on the label), or cooked bok choy, turnip greens, mustard greens, or collards. (If you prefer uncooked vegetables, just double the amount.)

Other foods provide more moderate amounts of calcium and regularly including them in your diet will further help ensure you're meeting your needs. These are cooked dried beans, almond butter, soaked almonds, soy nuts, broccoli, kale, okra, sweet potatoes, figs, navel oranges, corn tortillas, and blackstrap molasses.

Healthy bones also depend on vitamin D, "the sunshine vitamin." Although we can make vitamin D when skin is exposed to strong sunlight, many people don't make enough. The farther you live from the equator, the harder it is to make vitamin D, and it's not possible to make it during the winter months in many regions. The darker your skin is, the harder it is to make vitamin D, too, and for everyone, aging causes a decline in vitamin D production.

The bottom line is that many people need a dietary source of vitamin D, at least during the winter. Some types of fish provide vitamin D but not enough to meet our needs. Although you might think that cow's milk is a source of vitamin D, it has it only because it's fortified. Other foods fortified with this nutrient include breakfast cereals and many types of plant milks. The easiest way to get enough vitamin D is to take a supplement providing at least 600 IUs per day.

While calcium and vitamin D get most of the credit for keeping bones strong, other diet and lifestyle factors are just as important. Protein is vital for a healthy skeleton, so it's important to make sure you're including plenty of beans and other protein-rich foods in your diet. While nutritionists once believed that too much protein caused bones to lose calcium, more recent research shows that protein promotes a strong skeleton.

OUR LOVE AFFAIR WITH ANIMAL PROTEIN

For many years, nutrition scientists undervalued the protein in plants. Historically, the protein quality of different foods was assessed through studies in rats. It turned out that rats have different requirements than humans for amino acids, the building blocks of protein. Beans, for example, are not a great protein source for rats. But using more modern techniques to assess protein, researchers have found that these foods are perfectly fine as a protein source for humans. Those early animal studies have caused confusion and misinformation about protein for a long time.

In 1971, Frances Moore Lappé's book Diet for a Small Planet shed light on the harmful effects of animal agriculture on the planet (see page 33). It also laid out requirements for eating plant foods in certain combinations in order to meet amino acid needs. These recommendations made sense at the time, given the scientific understanding of protein nutrition. By the 1980s, it had become clear that this wasn't necessary and that meeting protein needs from plants was far easier than Lappé suggested. In the ten-year anniversary edition of the book, she corrected this misinformation. But so great is the love affair with meat that these erroneous ideas about plant protein have stuck in the consciousness of many.

Compounds in fruits and vegetables are also beneficial for bone health, and people who eat generous amounts of these foods often have the strongest bones. Exercise is another essential for strong, healthy bones.

Good-for-You Fats

Some of the healthiest diets in the world, like those that are traditional in countries around the Mediterranean Sea, are rich in plant fats. The fats found in nuts, seeds, avocadoes, and olives are good for you and so are the oils made from these foods. While oils should be used with a light hand, a teaspoon or two can go a long way toward enhancing flavors and can also improve absorption of nutrients and healthful plant compounds.

> **Every time you replace an animal food with a plant-based choice, you have an impact.**

It's important to make sure you include foods in your diet that provide the essential omega-3 fatty acids. To make sure you're meeting needs, include a small serving (a tablespoon or so) of ground flaxseeds, chopped walnuts, chia seeds, or 1 tablespoon of walnut or canola oil or a couple of teaspoons of flaxseed or hempseed oil in your daily consumption.

While you absolutely need the omega-3 fat found in flaxseed, walnuts, and canola oil, there is another family of omega-3 fats that is not considered essential. These are the fats found in fatty fish and in fish oil supplements. We talked a little bit about these fats, which are called DHA and EPA, in chapter 7 because they may be helpful in countering some types of depression and may also reduce risk for other chronic diseases. The scientific jury is out on whether there is any benefit to taking supplements of DHA and EPA. But if you wish to include them in your diet, choose a supplement that gets DHA and EPA from microalgae rather than fish. These vegan supplements are better for animals and better for the environment.

Vitamin B12

You may have heard that vitamin B12 is a big issue in vegan nutrition. It is, but it's not an issue that is exclusive to vegans. Animal foods are the only natural sources of this vitamin since B12 doesn't occur naturally in plants. Contrary to popular belief, you cannot get vitamin B12 from fermented foods, sea vegetables, or organic vegetables. But because even meat-eaters are advised to limit consumption of animal foods and to emphasize plant foods, anyone who is trying to eat more healthfully could fall short of meeting vitamin B12 needs. Also, as people age, it becomes more difficult to absorb the vitamin B12 that occurs naturally in foods. Vitamin B12 is far easier to absorb from supplements and fortified foods. Medical professionals advise everyone over the age of fifty, no matter how much meat they eat, to take a B12 supplement or include B12-fortified foods in their diet. So whether you are vegan, taking steps toward being more vegan, striving to eat healthfully, or are over fifty, you need to give some attention to vitamin B12.

The consequences of inadequate vitamin B12 can be serious, but getting enough is about the simplest thing in the world.

Humans have complex processes in place to manage vitamin B12 absorption: the less often you take it, the more you need. So the dosage recommendations for supplements may look unusual, but they make sense given our biology.

To make sure you're getting enough vitamin B12, do any one of the following:

- Take a daily supplement providing 25 to 100 micrograms of vitamin B12 in the cyanocobalamin form.

- Take a supplement of 1,000 micrograms twice per week.

- Eat two or three servings per day of foods that are fortified with this nutrient. Many plant milks have vitamin B12 added. Breakfast cereals often have it as well. If you use nutritional yeast on a regular basis, choose one that is grown on a vitamin B12-rich medium. The one that is most commonly available is made by Red Star and is labeled Vegetarian Support Formula. Note that neither brewer's yeast nor the active yeast used in baking is a source of vitamin B12.

A Shake of (Iodized) Salt

Iodine, a mineral that's needed for healthy metabolism, is difficult to measure in diets because the iodine content of foods varies depending on where the food is grown and how much iodine is in the soil. Food grown along coastal areas is likely to be higher in iodine, but that's a difficult thing to track when you're choosing vegetables in the grocery store.

Dairy foods are a reliable source of iodine but only because it's in the feed given to the cows and also in cleaning solutions used on dairy farms. Iodine from those cleaning solutions can leach into milk—which doesn't seem like a very appetizing way to get nutrients.

The easiest way to make sure you're getting iodine is to choose iodized salt. You don't want to overdo it with salt, of course, but just a few shakes every day will help you meet your iodine needs. Sea salt is usually not iodized and isn't a reliable source of this mineral.

Iron and Zinc

When you think of iron, foods like liver and red meat most likely come to mind. But plant foods are packed with iron. A serving of a plant protein source like lentils and black beans gives you about twice the amount of iron as a serving of red meat. Other foods that are rich in iron include whole grains, leafy green vegetables, sea vegetables, dried fruit, and soyfoods.

It's important for vegans to eat vitamin C-rich foods along with foods that provide iron. Vitamin C helps the body absorb the iron in plant foods. This does not require a lot of planning; it's likely that you do this often without knowing it. Whole grains, beans, and soyfoods are all good sources of iron. The best sources of vitamin C are peppers,

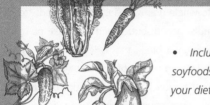

• Include legumes—beans, soyfoods, and peanuts—in your diet every day.

• Choose at least two cups per day of calcium-rich foods like forti-fied plant milks and juices, tofu made with calcium-sulfate, cooked bok choy, turnip greens, mustard greens, or collards.

• Take regular supplements of vitamin D and vitamin B12. Consider a supplement of the omega-3 fats DHA and EPA, too.

• Use a little bit of iodized salt on your food (just a few shakes).

• Choose whole grains over refined as often as possible.

• Include nuts or seeds in your diet, especially the ones that provide omega-3 fats such as walnuts, flaxseed, and hempseed.

• Eat plenty of fruits and vegetables, and include the ones that are rich in vitamin C as often as possible.

broccoli, cabbage, brussels sprouts, cauliflower, guava, papaya, kiwi-fruit, oranges, strawberries, pineapple, grapefruit, and cantaloupe. When you eat oatmeal topped with strawberries, stir-fried tofu with broccoli, or peppers stuffed with brown rice, you're taking advantage of vitamin C to improve iron absorption.

The same foods that give you plenty of iron also offer a generous dose of zinc. In addition to whole grains, beans, and soyfoods, foods that provide zinc include nuts, peanut butter, and seeds like pumpkin and sunflower seeds. Whole-grain bread that is leavened with yeast or sourdough is an especially good source of zinc since the leavening improves absorption. The best approach to getting enough of this nutrient is to choose whole grains over refined (always a good idea no matter what), include plenty of beans and soyfoods in your diet, and eat a couple servings of nuts and seeds every day.

Eat the Rainbow

Fruits and vegetables are nutritional powerhouses, and they are also packed with antioxidants and other plant compounds that are linked to a lower risk for chronic illnesses. For people eating mostly plant foods, they provide a couple of other benefits. We've already seen that the vitamin C in these foods helps with iron absorption. And the vegetables that boast bright yellow, orange, and green pigments are a source of vitamin A for vegans. The best sources are leafy greens like spinach, Swiss chard, winter squash, carrots, pumpkin, and sweet potatoes. Cantaloupe and papaya are also good sources of these vitamin A provitamins.

MOVING FORWARD

By this point, you may have found a brand or two of plant milk and non-dairy cheese that you like. Maybe you've tried our recipe for barbecued jackfruit or have discovered how remarkably good veggie burgers can be. You may have successfully baked a cake without eggs and explored options for introducing more beans into your diet.

If you're interested in shifting ever closer to a vegan diet, this kind of experimenting is a tried-and-true approach. Research shows that people who make the transition in a one-step-at-a-time fashion tend to be most successful in maintaining changes for the long term. This goes for all types of behavior change, not just adopting a vegan lifestyle.

While we've emphasized food choices in this book, the scope of veganism is far greater than what is on your plate. Your purchasing habits provide you with all types of opportunities to express a commitment to justice, compassion, fairness, and inclusiveness. Choosing clothing that is not made with animal skins or fibers and that is not produced in conditions that exploit humans is an important vegan practice. We don't have the choice yet to buy medicines that are free of animal testing, but we can seek out cruelty-free personal care products. These are readily available in grocery stores and drugstores. We can also opt for

> **Your purchasing habits provide you with opportunities to express a commitment to justice, compassion, fairness, and inclusiveness**

entertainment that doesn't exploit animals, like sanctuaries instead of zoos and aquariums or circuses that highlight incredible performances by talented humans instead of forced tricks by abused animals.

In this last set of daily actions, we offer two "recipes" for making your own cruelty-free and very frugal cleaning supplies. We also offer guidance to help you find vegan food when you're out and about and to establish a plan that will make vegan meals second nature. Finally, we offer a bonus daily action: it is always fun to celebrate together, and a Vegan Resistance Meal may be just the thing!

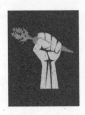

Daily Action 27:

MAKE YOUR OWN CLEANING SUPPLIES TO AVOID ONES TESTED ON ANIMALS

It takes just a minute or two to make your own furniture polish, saving you money and animals from the cruelty of animal testing.

Lemon Oil Furniture Polish

2 tablespoons fresh lemon juice

2–3 drops lemon oil

2–3 drops olive or jojoba oil

Combine the ingredients and use by dipping a clean cloth into the mix and rubbing onto wood furniture.

All-Purpose Surface Cleaner

1 cup water

1 tablespoon cruelty-free dish soap liquid

10 drops tea tree oil

Combine the ingredients in a large spray bottle. Use to clean kitchen and bathroom surfaces.

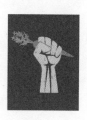

Daily Action 28:

PLAN A VEGAN MEAL FOR YOUR NEXT TRIP OR EVENING OUT

If you're an urban dweller or you live in a college town, you probably have plenty of vegan options when you're out and about. Even in those cases, though, you may find yourself at a business or social event at a steak house or traveling in areas where you can't find vegan restaurants. Unless you are happy with meals of salad and French fries, you may need to get a little bit creative.

If you have a choice of restaurants, look for ones that serve Indian, Middle Eastern, Mexican, Thai, Chinese, or Ethiopian cuisine. You will almost always find vegan options at these restaurants without asking for any special preparation (although, at most Mexican restaurants, you'll need to ask the server to substitute guacamole for the cheese and sour cream). Some fast-food southwestern-style eateries like Chipotle, Moe's Southwest Grill, and Hot Harry's even offer tofu—which may be a little unusual for this style of eating, but makes a surprisingly good taco bowl or burrito.

For casual dining, you can find vegan veggie burgers at a surprising number of popular restaurants, like White Castle, Denny's, and Red Robin. We recommend downloading the HappyCow app onto your phone for a list of restaurants with vegan and vegetarian offerings in cities and towns all over the United States.

But what if you find yourself at a restaurant where there is not one vegan entrée on the menu? In that case, you'll need to build your own. Start with something filling and substantial like pasta or a baked potato. Then do a thorough investigation of the menu looking for ingredients that the chef can add to the pasta. These items may be among the menu's side dishes, but they might also be components of entrées. Look for grilled portobello mushrooms, sautéed onions, and roasted vegetables. An Italian restaurant that serves homemade minestrone will have beans on hand. A steak house might have beans among its salad bar offerings. Ask to have them incorporated into your pasta dish (or grab them from the salad bar yourself) to create a more substantial entrée.

When you're headed out on a road trip, highway rest stops are great for grabbing coffee and soft drinks, but they rarely offer much more in the way of food than burgers, pizza, and cinnamon rolls. Bring a cooler and stock it with vegan cheese and crackers, mixed nuts, apples and peanut butter, sandwiches of vegan deli slices with pickles and mustard. For something hot, bring a thermos of soup. Instant oatmeal and small cartons of shelf-stable plant milks make a fast, healthy breakfast in your hotel room. Stir in a vegan protein powder or peanut butter powder for a protein boost.

Nut butter on crackers, trail mix, and instant soup cups are also good snacks for long plane flights. It's increasingly easy to find vegan food at airports, too. Food courts usually have burritos or Chinese stir-fried dishes. Look, too, for Cibo Express gourmet markets, which are commonly found in major airports in the US and always have interesting vegan options.

Daily Action 29:

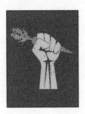

"VEGANIZE" FIVE FAVORITE RECIPES

It takes just a few tricks to transform almost any favorite recipe into its vegan version. The key is to pay attention to texture and flavor while taking advantage of tried-and-true substitutions.

In chapter 4 you learned how easy it is to capture the essence of umami and in chapter 2, the options for finding smoky flavors of processed meats like bacon and sausage with ingredients like liquid smoke and smoked paprika.

To capture the creamy textures often associated with dairy foods, use whipped, full-fat coconut milk, blended soft tofu, or soaked, pureed cashews. Commercial vegan sour cream and cream cheese come in handy for these purposes, too. And yes, there is wonderful vegan ice

VEGAN WITH A FEW TWEAKS
HOW TO VEGANIZE (ALMOST) ANYTHING

Instead of . . .	Try a commercial substitute	Or make your own!
Cow's milk	Any kind of plant milk	
Butter	Vegan butter, oil, coconut oil	
Cheese	Commercial cream cheese, cheddar, mozzarella, and more	Soaked cashews or macadamia nuts blended with oil, miso, salt, and herbs
Cream	Vegan whipped cream or dessert topping, sour cream, coffee creamer	• Skim the top portion from a can of culinary full-fat coconut milk and whip it with a beater until thick. • Blend soft silken tofu in a blender or food processor. • Soak raw cashews for two hours and then blend with a little bit of water until creamy. • ¾ cup + 1 tablespoon soy milk and 3 tablespoons melted vegan butter or coconut oil replaces a cup of cream.
Eggs for baking	Egg replacer powder Soy flour	Aquafaba Flaxseed powder
Ham or bacon in soups and beans	Liquid smoke, smoked paprika, imitation bacon bits, commercial tempeh bacon	
Chicken broth	Bouillon cubes or powder	Homemade vegetable stock
Buttermilk		2 teaspoons vinegar stirred into 1 cup soy milk. Let stand until separated.
Any meat	Look for vegan chicken strips, chicken nuggets, sausages, beef cubes and ground beef, crab cakes, breaded fish fillets, bacon, and more.	Freeze tofu in its container (not silken tofu, but tofu in water). Defrost, squeeze out the liquid it absorbed, but don't squeeze so energetically that it loses all its liquid! With your fingers, shred it, sauté it for a few minutes, and then substitute it for beef in sloppy joes or tomato sauce.

cream. Even Ben and Jerry's makes nondairy versions of some of their popular flavors.

A chewy, meaty texture can come from frozen tofu, soy curls, and the vast array of veggie meats in the grocery—everything from burgers to crab cakes, all made from plants.

Happily, most of your favorite condiments are naturally vegan. Ketchup, mustard, pickles, salsa, relish, barbecue sauce, tapenade, balsamic vinegar, roasted peppers, sun-dried tomatoes—you'll find all of these items in the refrigerators of meat-eaters and vegans alike.

You can also find vegan versions of nonvegan items like mayonnaise and Worcestershire sauce.

As you become more familiar with all of these foods and ingredients, it gets easy to find new recipes and to revamp old ones to make them vegan. Our "How to Veganize Anything" chart summarizes some of the tricks and tips we've talked about throughout the book as well as some additional ideas.

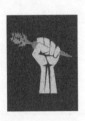

Daily Action 30:
MAKE A MENU PLAN

New habits don't just happen; you need a plan. No matter how committed you are to making something vegan for dinner, it's going to be tough if the only things in your refrigerator are ground beef, eggs, and last night's leftover macaroni and cheese. Stock your pantry with beans, including canned beans, soy curls, TVP, whole grains and pasta, favorite vegan cereals, and all the condiments you love to use in your cooking. Keep favorite veggie meats and other convenience products in the freezer for those days when you need a fast meal. Keep a selection of nuts and seeds in the refrigerator.

If you love to cook, it can be fun to have a file filled with recipes. But most people have less variety in their diets than you might think. We tend to eat the same three or four things for breakfast, the same selection of soups, salads, and sandwiches for lunch, and maybe eight or ten different menus for dinner. Once you realize that, it becomes much easier to come up with a plan for vegan options. Make a list of ten vegan dinners you think you'll enjoy or already enjoy, and maybe three or four breakfasts, lunches, and snacks. Stock your pantry with the foods you need for those meals and you are set. It truly is that easy.

Bonus Daily Action:

HOST A COMMUNAL RESISTANCE DINNER

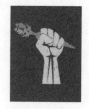

Thank you to Carol's sister Nancy for inspiring us to explore ideas for recipes for a Resistance Feast. We present two ideas for feasts, one featuring Trumped Up Vegan Cutlets a L'Orange and the other featuring a Stop the Wall Taco Salad with Fire and Fury Salsa. We asked vegan chef Bryanna Clark Grogan to help us devise some of the recipes. Bryanna has devoted over fifty years to the study of cooking and nutrition and is the author of eight vegan cookbooks, including *World Vegan Feast*. She blogs at *veganfeastkitchen.blogspot.ca*.

Resistance Feast 1

Drain the Swamp Kitchen Cabinet Compote
Trumped Up Vegan Cutlets a L'Orange
Tiny Little Chocolate-Nut-Cherry Thumbprint Candies

Drain the Swamp Kitchen Cabinet Compote

Makes 4–6 servings

This recipe comes from Carol's sister Nancy Adams, and it's a good way to use up spoiling or freezer-burned fruits. Nancy says of the recipe: "Rhubarb, overripe bananas, and overripe apples, sugar to taste—looks quite swampy, but tastes great!" Here is one way to drain the swamp, but you can do so using whatever fruit you have on hand.

    1 pound rhubarb
    2 (mostly bad) apples with the rot cut out
    2 overripe bananas, not yet black
    2 cups apple cider
    ¼ cup sugar

- Simmer the rhubarb, apples, and bananas in the cider until the rhubarb is soft. Add the sugar, taste, and add more if needed.

- Serve with vegan yogurt or sour cream.

Trumped Up Vegan Cutlets à L'Orange

By Bryanna Clark Grogan
Serves 4

This recipe doesn't look like the classic one, you say? Of course not! It's the "Trumped-Up" version. If you are using breaded chicken cutlets like those made by Boca, skip the first five ingredients.

Seasoned coating for dredging:
    2 cups whole-wheat flour
    ¼ cup nutritional yeast flakes
    1 teaspoon salt

1 teaspoon onion powder

Optional: 1 teaspoon garlic granules or powder

4 large vegan cutlets such as Gardein Lightly Seasoned Chick'n
   Scallopini

3 large oranges

1 cup vegan "chicken-y" broth

½ cup vegan "beef-y" broth

½ cup water

2 tablespoons brown sugar

1 tablespoon cornstarch or wheat starch (Do not substitute other
   starches.)

3 tablespoons dry to medium sherry

2 tablespoons vegan butter

Salt and freshly ground black pepper to taste

Olive oil

- If using uncoated chicken cutlets, combine the whole wheat flour, nutritional yeast flakes, salt, onion powder, and optional garlic powder. Place some of the flour mixture in a shallow bowl and dredge the cutlets. Set aside.

- Wash and dry the oranges. Grate the orange part of the rind of one orange. Peel the orange part of the rind of the second orange with a fruit peeler and set it aside. Juice the third orange and set the juice aside.

- Carefully trim the white pith off of both peeled oranges and slice into ½ inch slices. Cut the slices in half.

- In a medium saucepan, mix together the broths, water, and brown sugar. Bring to a boil over high heat. Add the strips of orange peel and the orange juice. Reduce heat and simmer uncovered for 10 to 15 minutes.

- Whisk the cornstarch with the sherry and stir into the simmering sauce. Stir briefly until it thickens. Taste and season with salt and pepper. Strain the sauce to remove the orange peel. Stir in the vegan butter until it melts. Pour back into the saucepan and add some of the orange slices.

- Heat a tablespoon of oil in a large skillet and brown the seasoned cutlets until crispy and lightly browned.

- Place the cutlets on a serving platter and drizzle with a generous amount of the orange sauce. Sprinkle with grated zest and garnish with the remaining orange slices. Serve with baked or mashed potatoes, a tossed salad, and warm bread.

Tiny Little Chocolate-Nut-Cherry Thumbprint Candies

By Bryanna Clark Grogan
Makes about 45–48 small candies

Your dinner guests will be impressed by these fancy little candies that are deceptively easy to make.

> 2 cups vegan semisweet chocolate chips
> 1 cup nut butter
> 3 tablespoons refined coconut oil
> 2 tablespoons maple syrup
> 1 cup chopped roasted nuts (same variety as the nut butter)—
>   they can be salted, if you like
> Optional 2 teaspoons vanilla extract
> Filling: about 1 cup of commercial or homemade cherry jam or
>   preserves

- Place the chocolate chips, nut butter, coconut oil, and syrup in the top of a double boiler over simmering water. When the mixture can be mixed together smoothly, stir in the nuts (and optional vanilla, if using) until the nuts are well-distributed throughout the mixture.

- Let cool enough so that the mixture is firm enough to not stick to your fingers, but is still pliable. Drop the mixture by heaping teaspoonfuls on parchment-covered baking sheets. Immediately press a thumbprint indentation into the center of each spoonful, then gently press together any cracked edges.

- Fill each indentation with about ½ teaspoon of the cherry jam or preserves—don't overfill. Place the baking sheets in the refrigerator until they are quite firm. Then they can be stored in the refrigerator or freezer in storage containers with tight lids with baking parchment between layers.

Resistance Feast 2

"Stop The Wall" Taco Salad Bowl with Fire and Fury Salsa
imPeach Crumble

"Stop the Wall" Taco Salad Bowl with Fire and Fury Salsa

By Bryanna Clark Grogan
Serves 4

Canned chipotle peppers in adobo sauce (chipotle chiles en adobo) are smoked, dried jalapeño peppers canned in a tangy red sauce and easily available in most supermarkets. They add not only heat, but also a pleasant smokiness to the salsa.

   1 cup thawed, frozen sweet corn kernels, drained
   2 medium ripe tomatoes, chopped (or about 2 cups chopped
      grape tomatoes)
   ½ cup chopped red onion

½ cup sliced pitted black or kalamata olives

1 medium green pepper, trimmed and chopped

2 chopped canned chipotle peppers in adobo sauce, or more, according to your taste

1 tablespoon lime juice

1 teaspoon ground cumin

½ teaspoon salt

Optional 1 tablespoon or more minced fresh cilantro (parsley if you don't like cilantro)

4 cups rinsed and drained cooked or canned pinto beans or black beans

1 tablespoon taco seasoning or chili paste

4 large whole-grain "tortilla bowls" (sometimes called "tostada bowls" or "taco bowls") purchased or homemade from 10-inch tortillas (see instructions in the recipe)

Sliced crisp lettuce

4 cups hot cooked quinoa or brown rice

Toppings: (use one, two, or all three)

Sliced ripe avocado brushed with fresh lemon juice

Vegan sour cream

Shredded vegan white cheese

- Make the salsa by combining the corn, tomatoes, onion, olives, green pepper, chipotle peppers, lime juice, cumin, salt, and optional cilantro. Refrigerate until serving time.

- Stir the taco seasoning or chili paste into the beans and set aside.

- If you are making your own tortilla bowls, preheat the oven to 425 degrees. Spray or brush both sides of the tortillas with oil and drape each one over a small oven safe soup bowl. Place the soup bowls on a baking sheet. Bake until crisp, 10 to 15 minutes, rotating the baking sheets halfway through. Let them cool completely before removing from the bowls or pans.

- To assemble the taco bowls, line the inside of each tortilla bowl with a ring of crisp sliced lettuce. Place a scoop of hot cooked rice or quinoa in the center of the tortilla bowl. Top with a good portion of the beans and then a generous portion of the salsa. Serve with bowls of avocado, vegan sour cream, and shredded lettuce on the side.

imPeach Crumble

Makes 12 servings

Most cake mixes are vegan, but be sure to check the label. This recipe uses a handy trick—replacing the eggs and oil that cake mixes call for with a can of soda or seltzer.

1 pound frozen peach slices, defrosted
1 box vanilla cake mix
12 ounces club soda
½ cup chopped walnuts

- Preheat the oven according to package directions on the cake mix.

- Spread the peaches over the bottom of a 9-by-13-inch nonstick cake pan.

- Pour the cake mix into a mixing bowl. Pour the club soda over the mix and stir quickly to combine. Make sure the cake mix is all moistened but don't overmix.

- Pour the batter over the peaches. Sprinkle the top with the walnuts. Bake according to package directions. You may need to give this cake an extra 3 or 4 minutes to cook through.

* * * * * *

When you choose a plant-based diet, you're doing good in a myriad of ways *at once*. And, as we suggested at the beginning of this book, what happens in the kitchen doesn't stay in the kitchen. We hope you will bring the ideas, insights, and ingredients you have learned about from this book into your everyday resistance. During a time when you may feel disempowered, your food choices can be a source of empowerment. Our lives *are* meaningful against injustice as every day we make meaningful choices. Veganism offers a daily way to enact your values, while helping to protect the environment, to challenge misogyny and other oppressive attitudes, to cultivate compassion, and to enhance your health. Acting as individuals in decisions about our daily food choices is not immaterial; it is an essential part of resistance.

What happens in the kitchen doesn't stay in the kitchen . . .

What's in your protest kitchen?

RECOMMENDED RESOURCES

VEGANISM AND SOCIAL JUSTICE

Adams, Carol J. *The Sexual Politics of Meat*. Bloomsbury, 2015.

Adams, Carol J., and Lori Gruen, eds. *Ecofeminism: Feminist Intersections with Other Animals and the Earth*. Bloomsbury, 2014.

"{Bio}graphies" series from Lantern Books, including:

- pattrice jones, *The Oxen at the Intersection: A Collision*

- Alex Lockword, *The Pig in Thin Air: An Identification*

- Martin Rowe, *The Elephants in the Room: An Excavation and The Polar Bar in the Zoo: A Speculation*

Brueck, Julia Feliz, ed. *Veganism in an Oppressive World: A Vegans-of-Color Community Project*. Sanctuary Publishers, 2017.

Harper, Breeze, ed. *Sistah Vegan: Black Female Vegans Speak out on Food, Identity, Health and Society*. Lantern Books, 2010.

Hawthorne, Mark. *A Vegan Ethic: Embracing a Life of Compassion for All*. Changemakers Books, 2016.

jones, pattrice. *After Shock: Confronting Trauma in a Violent World: A Guide for Activists and their Allies*. Lantern Books, 2007.

Kim, Claire Jean. *Dangerous Crossings: Race, Species, and Nature in a Multicultural Age*. Cambridge University Press, 2015.

Ko, Aph, and Syl Ko. *Aphro-ism: Essays on Pop Culture, Feminism, and Black Veganism from Two Sisters*. Lantern Books, 2017.

Nibert, David. *Animal Rights, Human Rights: Entanglements of Oppression and Liberation*. Rowman & Littlefield, 2002.

Taylor, Sunaura. *Beasts of Burden: Animal and Disability Liberation*. The New Press, 2017.

NUTRITION RESOURCES

www.vegan.com/nutrition

www.veganhealth.org

www.vegetariannutrition.net

Brueck, Julia Feliz. *Baby and Toddler Vegan Feeding Guide*. Sanctuary Publishers, 2017.

Davis, Brenda, and Vesanto Melina. *Becoming Vegan*. Book Publishing Company, 2013.

Mangels, Reed. *The Everything Vegan Pregnancy Book*. Adams Media, 2011.

Messina, Virginia, and JL Fields. *Vegan for Her*. Da Capo Press, 2013.

Norris, Jack, and Virginia Messina. *Vegan for Life*. Da Capo Press, 2011.

Rebhal, Sayward. *Vegan Pregnancy Survival Guide*. Herbivore Books, 2011.

Wasserman, Debra, and Reed Mangels. *Simply Vegan*, fourth edition. The Vegetarian Resource Group, 2006.

VEGAN LIFESTYLE

Cruelty-free apps:

- Bunny Free

- Leaping Bunny

- Cruelty Cutter

Adams, Carol J. *Living Among Meat Eaters: The Vegetarian's Survival Handbook*. Lantern, 2010.

ONLINE STORES

www.cosmosveganshoppe.com
www.herbivoreclothing.com
www.veganessentials.com
www.thevegetariansite.com

COOKBOOKS

Atlas, Nava. *Wild About Greens*. Sterling, 2012.

Ciment, Ethan, and Michael Suchman. *NYC Vegan*. Vegan Heritage Press, 2017.

Costigan, Fran. *Vegan Chocolate: Unapologetically Luscious and Decadent Dairy-Free Desserts*. Running Press, 2013.

Fields, JL. *Vegan Pressure Cooking*. Fair Winds Press, 2015.

Garza, Eddie. *Salud! Vegan Mexican Cookbook*. Rockridge Press, 2016.

Grogan, Bryanna Clark. *World Vegan Feast*. Vegan Heritage Press, 2011.

Hamshaw, Gena. *Power Plates*. Ten Speed Press, 2018.

Hasson, Julie. *Vegan Diner*. Running Press, 2011.

Hester, Kathy. *The Vegan Slow Cooker*. Fair Winds, 2011.

Hingle, Richa. *Vegan Richa's Indian Kitchen*. Vegan Heritage Press, 2015.

Romero, Terry Hope. *Vegan Eats World*. Da Capo Lifelong Books, 2012

Schinner, Miyoko. *The Homemade Vegan Pantry*. Ten Speed Press, 2015.

Schwegmann, Michelle, and Josh Hooten. *Eat Like You Give a Damn*. Book Publishing Company, 2015.

Shannon, Annie and Dan. *Mastering the Art of Vegan Cooking*. Grand Central Lifestyle. 2015.

Simpson, Alicia. *Vegan Comfort Food*. The Experiment, 2009.

Terry, Bryant. *Afro-Vegan*. Ten Speed Press, 2014.

SOURCES

CHAPTER 1

p. 8. Two-thirds of Democrats…Betsy Cooper, Daniel Cox, Rachel Lienesch, Robert P. Jones, "The Divide Over America's Future: 1950 or 2050?" 10.25.2016. *www. prri.org/research/poll-1950s-2050-divided-nations-direction-post-election/*.

p. 8. Violent responses to African American attempts to integrate the suburbs. Richard Rothstein, *The Color of Law: A Forgotten History of How Our Government Segregated America*. New York: Liveright, 2017, p. 147.

p. 9. The diet of pre-Conquest Mesoamericans: Luz Calvo and Catriona Rueda Esquibel, *Decolonize Your Diet: Plant-Based Mexican-American Recipes for Health and Healing*. Vancouver: Arsenal Pulp Press, 2017.

p. 9. The diffusion of African dietary preferences, including the hiding of rice: Judith A. Carney and Richard Nicholas Rosomoff, *In the Shadow of Slavery: Africa's Botanical Legacy in the Atlantic World*. Berkeley and Los Angeles: University of California Press, 2009, p. 76.

p. 9. West African foodways, *In the Shadow of Slavery*, p. 91.

p. 11. George Beard, M.D., *Sexual Neurasthenia: Its Hygiene, Causes, Symptoms and Treatment with a Chapter on Diet for the Nervous*. New York: E. B. Treat & Co., 1898, pp. 272–78.

p. 11. "Hooved locusts," Jeremy Rifkin, *Beyond Beef: The Rise and Fall of the Cattle Culture*. New York: Dutton Books, 1992, pp. 200–12.

p. 12. *Hog Management* quoted in Jim Mason and Peter Singer, *Animal Factories*. New York: Crown, 1981, p. 1.

p. 12. The sow as a piece of machinery, quoted in C. David Coats, *Old MacDonald's Factory Farm*. New York: Continuum Books, 1989, p. 32.

p. 12. The modern layer as a converting machine, quoted in Ruth Harrison, *Animal Machines*. Oxfordshire and Boston: CABI, 2013 (reprint of 1964 edition), p. 75.

p. 14. Strange noises turn out to be cows missing their calves, *http://www.newburyportnews.com/news/local_news/strange-noises-turn-out-to-be-cows-missing-their-calves/article_d872e4da-b318-5e90-870e-51266f8eea7f.html.*

p. 14. Racially explicit laws created urban ghettos and white suburbs: Rothstein, *The Color of Law*, p. xii.

p. 15. Stephanie Coontz on the "collapse" of traditional family values. *The Way We Never Were: American Families and the Nostalgia Trap*. New York: Basic Books, 1992/2016, p. 56.

pp. 16–17. Information on the Animal Enterprise Terrorism Act, Will Potter, *Green is the New Red*. San Francisco: City Lights, 2011.

p. 18. Amount of time women spent doing housework, *The Way We Were*, Coontz, p. 28.

CHAPTER 2

p. 30. Increase in record highs due to global warming, Meehl GA, et al., Relative increase of record high maximum temperatures compared to record low minimum temperatures in the U.S. *Geophys Res Lett*. 2009: 36.

p. 30. NASA scientists' estimates about rise in temperatures, *https://earthobservatory.nasa.gov/Features/GlobalWarming/page5.php.*

p. 30. Great Barrier Reef, T.P. Hughes et al., "Global warming and recurrent mass bleaching of corals." *Nature*. 2017; 543: 373–7.

p. 30 Loss of sea ice, C Parmesan, "Ecological and evolutionary responses to recent climate change," *Annu Rev Ecol Evol Syst*. 2006; 37: 637–69.

p. 31. Kristin Laidre on polar bears, *https://climate.nasa.gov/news/2499/polar-bears-across-the-arctic-face-shorter-sea-ice-season.*

p. 31. Interaction among plants, animals, insects and bacteria, *http://www.ipsnews.net/2007/05/biodiversity-scientists-foresee-extinction-domino-effect.*

p. 32. Glacier mass and melt, G.A. Meehl et al., "Global climate projections," in *Climate Change 2007: The Physical Basis. Contribution of Working Group I to the Fourth Assessment Report of the Intergovernmental Panel on Climate Change*. Cambridge and New York: Cambridge University Press, pp. 747–845.

p. 32. Decrease of eight major crops, J. Knox, "Climate change impacts on crop productivity in Africa and South Asia." *Environ Res Lett* 2012; 7.

p. 32 Obama White House memorandum on climate change, *https:// obamawhitehouse.archives.gov/the-press-office/2016/09/21/ presidential-memorandum-climate-change-and-national-security.*

p. 32 Climate change and terrorism, *https://www.newclimateforpeace.org/ blog/insurgency-terrorism-and-organised-crime-warming-climate.*

p. 33. Climate justice and disability, *http://www.newmobility.com/2016/03/ climate-change-and-disability.*

p. 33. Frances Moore Lappé, *Diet for a Small Planet.* New York: Ballantine Books, 1971.

p. 34. Animal protein versus soy protein resource use, L. Reijnders, S. Soret, "Quantification of the environmental impact of different dietary protein choices." *Am J Clin Nutr.* 2003; 78: 664S–8S.

p. 34. Meat-eaters' diets required more water and fertilizer, H. J. Marlow et al., "Diet and the environment: does what you eat matter?" *Am J Clin Nutr* 2009; 89: 1699S–1703S.

p. 34. Statistics on animal waste, L. Horrigan et al., "How sustainable agriculture can address the environmental and human health harms of industrial agriculture." *Environ Health Perspect.* 2002; 110: 445–56.

p. 34. Impact of untreated waste, A.Z. Akhtar et al., "Health professionals' roles in animal agriculture, climate change, and human health." *Am J Prev Med* 2009; 36: 182–7.

pp. 34–35. Chemical runoff from factory farms, J. Sabate, S. Soret, "Sustainability of plant-based diets: back to the future." *Am J Clin Nutr* 2014; 100 Suppl 1: 476S–82S.

p. 35. Marine ecologist Daniel Pauly quote, *https://newrepublic.com/ article/69712/aquacalypse-now.*

p. 35. Wasted energy from farming shrimp and salmon, S.S. De Silva, D. Soto, "Climate change and aquaculture: potential impacts, adaptation and mitigation." In K. Cochrane, C. De Young, D. Soto and T. Bahri (eds). "Climate change implications for fisheries and aquaculture: overview of current scientific knowledge." FAO Fisheries and Aquaculture Technical Paper. No. 530. Rome, FAO, 2009, pp. 151–212.

p. 35. Over-fishing of large carnivorous fish, E.K.A. Spiers et al., "Potential role of predators on carbon dynamics of marine ecosystems as assessed by a Bayesian belief network." *Ecological Informatics* 2016: 77–83.

p. 35. Food system and greenhouse gas emissions, S. J. Vermeulen et al., "Climate change and food systems." *Annu Rev Environ Resour* 2012; 37: 195–222; F.N. Tubiello et al., (2014), "Agriculture, Forestry and Other Land Use Emissions by Sources and Removals by Sinks: 1990–2011 Analysis" (FAO Statistics Division, Rome).

p. 35. Greenhouse gas emissions of meat, dairy products, M. Berners-Lee et al., "The relative greenhouse gas impacts of realistic dietary choices." *Energy Policy* 2012; 43: 184–90.

p. 36 Greenhouse gas emissions based on dietary choices, P. Scarborough et al., "Dietary greenhouse gas emissions of meat-eaters, fish-eaters, vegetarians and vegans in the UK." *Clim Change* 2014; 125: 179–92.

p. 36 Greenhouse gas emissions and soyfood production, A. Mejia et al., "Greenhouse gas emissions generated by tofu production: A case study." *J Hunger Environmental* Nutr. 2017; Hoekstra AY, The water footprint of animal products, in: D'Silva J, Webster J, eds. *The Meat Crisis: Developing More Sustainable Production and Consumption*. London, UK: Earthscan, 2010; 22–33.

p. 37. Substituting beans for beef, H. Harwatt et al., "Substituting beans for beef as a contribution toward US climate change targets." *Climatic Change* 2017; 143: 261.

p. 37. Increased meat consumption, *http://www.worldwatch.org/global-meat-production-and-consumption-continue-rise*.

p. 41. Soy can have estrogenic and antiestrogenic effects. T. Oseni et al., "Selective estrogen receptor modulators and phytoestrogens." *Planta Med* 2008; 74: 1656–65.

p. 41. Consuming soyfoods and lower lifetime risk for breast cancer, L. A. Korde et al., "Childhood soy intake and breast cancer risk in Asian American women," *Cancer Epidemiol Biomarkers Prev* 2009; 18: 1050–9.

p. 41. Breast cancer survival and soy consumption, F. Chi et al., "Post-diagnosis soy food intake and breast cancer survival: A meta-analysis of cohort studies." *Asian Pacific Journal of Cancer Prevention* 2013; 14: 2407–12.

p. 41. Soy linked to lower risk for prostate cancer, C. C. Applegate et al., "Soy consumption and the risk of prostate cancer: An updated systematic review and meta-analysis." *Nutrients* 2018; 10.

p. 41. Cow's milk linked to increased risk for prostate cancer, D. Aune, D. A. Navarro Rosenblatt, D. S. Chan et al., "Dairy products, calcium, and prostate cancer risk: a systematic review and meta-analysis of cohort studies." *Am J Clin Nutr* 2015; 101: 87–117.

CHAPTER 3

p. 55. Food desert definition, *https://opinionator.blogs.nytimes.com /2012/04/25/time-to-revisit-food-deserts.*

p. 55. Small business funding, Chin Jou, *Super Sizing Urban America: How Inner Cities Got Fast Food with Government Help.* Chicago and London: The University of Chicago Press, 2017.

p. 55. Quotes from the Bureau of Animal Industry, "Hearings Before the Committee on Agriculture . . . on the So-called 'Beveridge Amendment' to the Agricultural Appropriation Bill," U.S. Congress, House, Committee on Agriculture, 1906, pp. 346–50, 59th Congress, 1st Session.

p. 56. Workers might make ten thousand cuts over a single shift, Jennifer Dillard, "Slaughterhouse Nightmares: Psychological Harm Suffered by Slaughterhouse Employees and the Possibility of Redress through Legal Reform." *Georgetown Journal on Poverty Law & Policy.* 15 (391).

p. 56. Rates of injury and illness among slaughterhouse workers, Michael S. Worrall, "Meatpacking Safety: Is OSHA Enforcement Adequate?" *Drake Journal of Agricultural.* Vol. 9.

p. 57. Psychological cost of slaughterhouse work, Dillard.

p. 57. Perpetration-induced stress disorder, Rachel McNair, "Perpetration-Induced Traumatic Stress: The Psychological Consequences of Killing," *Psychological Dimensions of War and Peace,* edited by Harvey Langholtz. New York: Authors Choice Press, 2005.

p. 57. Puerto Rican hurricane survivors, *http://www.omaha.com/eedition/sunrise/articles/far-from-home-puerto-ricans-begin-lives-they-never-imagined/article_cfb7d134-274e-5e1d-b0ab-b0cd285270ed.html.*

p. 57. Information on Christian Alcoholics & Addicts in Recovery (CAAIR), *https://www.currentaffairs.org/2017/12/why-isnt-this-a-major-national-scandal.*

pp. 57–58. Third-shift workers, *https://www.bloomberg.com/news/features/2017-12-29/america-s-worst-graveyard-shift-is-grinding-up-workers.*

p. 60. Urban garden in Milwaukee, WI, *https://civileats.com/2017/10/04/milwaukee-is-showing-how-urban-gardening-can-heal-a-city.*

CHAPTER 4

p. 71. The "Eat Like a Man" cover of *Muscle and Fitness* (June 2009), can be seen here: *https://www.amazon.com/MUSCLE-FITNESS-MAGAZINE-COVER-PHOTO/dp/B007QVTVC4/ref=sr_1_4?s=magazines&ie=UTF8&qid=1521855633&sr=8-4&keywords=muscle+and+fitness+eat+like+a+man.*

p. 71. "Testosterone wrapped in bacon," *Boston Globe* review, *https://www.bostonglobe.com/lifestyle/style/2016/06/06/flank-testosterone-wrapped-bacon-cutlery-optional/oBM1TdorZB6OsuoA6WY1HM/story.html.*

p. 71. The 2013 "Hurricane Doug" Taco Bell can be seen here: *https://www.adforum.com/creative-work/ad/player/34491786/hurricane-doug/taco-bell.*

p. 71. The Hummer ad and its original tagline "Restore your manhood" is discussed by Seth Stevenson, *http://www.slate.com/articles/business/ad_report_card/2006/08/suvs_for_hippies.html.*

p. 72. Soy effects on hormone status with excessively high intakes, J. Martinez, J.E. Lewi, "An unusual case of gynecomastia associated with soy product consumption." *Endocr Pract* 2008; 14: 415–8; T. Siepmann et al., "Hypogonadism and erectile dysfunction associated with soy product consumption," *Nutrition* 2011; 27: 859–62.

p. 72. Isoflavones do not impact testosterone levels, sperm count, or sperm quality, J. M Hamilton-Reeves et al., "Clinical studies show no effects of soy protein or isoflavones on reproductive hormones in men: results of a meta-analysis." *Fertil Steril* 2010; 94: 997–1007; M. Messina, "Soybean isoflavone exposure does not have feminizing effects on men: a critical examination of the clinical evidence." *Fertil Steril* 2010; 93: 2095–104; J. H. Mitchell et al., "Effect of a phytoestrogen food supplement on reproductive health in normal males." *Clin Sci (Lond)* 2001; 100: 613–8; L. K. Beaton et al., "Soy protein isolates of varying isoflavone content do not adversely affect semen quality in healthy young men," *Fertil Steril.* 2010; 94: 1717–22.

p. 72. Soy intake in Asia, M. Messina, C. Nagata, A. H. Wu, "Estimated Asian adult soy protein and isoflavone intakes." *Nutr Cancer* 2006; 55: 1–12.

p. 73. Rosie the Organic Chicken represents Petaluma Poultry. *https://www. petalumapoultry.com/products/rosie-organic.*

p. 74. The "KFC Hillary Special" button appears at minute 2:33 in a video from the *New York Times*, "Unfiltered Voices from Donald Trump's Crowds," August 3, 2016. *https://www.nytimes.com/video/us/politics/100000004533191/unfil tered-voices-from-donald-trumps-crowds.html.*

p. 74. Bridie Jabour, "Julia Gillard's 'small breasts' served up on Liberal party dinner menu." June 11, 2013. *https://www.theguardian.com/world/2013/ jun/12/gillard-menu-sexist-liberal-dinner.*

p 74. Saussie Pig BBQ image can be found here: *https://www.tripadvi sor.co.nz/LocationPhotoDirectLink–32416–d7265414–i120918938– The#Saussie#Pig–Fellsmere#Florida.html*

p. 74. The *Wikipedia* entry on "Breastaurants" refers to the double entendres in their names. Twin Peaks' ad campaign is referred to in Laura Shunk, "Twin Peaks brings beer, ballgames and boobs to Colorado Mills." October 11. 2011. *Westword. http://www.westword.com/restaurants/ twin-peaks-brings-beer-ballgames-and-boobs-to-colorado-mills-5765332.*

p. 75. One in five women in the United States has visited Planned Parenthood, Cecile Richards, Women's March on Washington, Jan. 21, 2017. Via live feed at the *New York Times* website. Accessed 1/21/2017.

p. 77. Dairy Air, *http://www.nj.com/entertainment/index.ssf/2017/12/dairy_ air_ice_cream_montclair_logo.html.*

p. 77. "Artificial insemination," *https://www.wikihow.com/Artificially -Inseminate-Cows-and-Heifers.*

p. 79. "pig roast." *https://slate.com/news-and-politics/2018/02/cornell-fra ternity-zeta-beta-tau-suspended-for-offensive-pig-roast-game.html.*

CHAPTER 5

p. 94. Alabama legislators, *https://www.nytimes.com/2017/12/11/ opinion/roy-moore-alabama-senate-voter-suppression.html?smid= tw-nytopinion&smtyp=cur.*

p. 94. The cop in Ferguson, MI, *http://theweek.com/speedreads/448306/ white-cop-calls-black-protesters-animals-ferguson-missouri.*

p. 94. Police officer Jennifer Lynne Silver referred on Instagram, *http:// photographyisnotacrime.com/2015/04/baltimore-county-cop-shuts-down- social-media-page-after-calling-freddie-gray-protesters-animals.*

p. 94. Kevin Young, *Bunk: The Rise of Hoaxes, Humbug, Plagiarists, Phonies, Post-Facts, and Fake News.* Minneapolis: Grey Wolf Press, 2017.

p. 95. "White by reputation in the community" replaced by "one-drop rule," Annette Gordon-Reed, *The Hemingses of Monticello: An American Family.* New York: W. W. Norton & Co., 2008, p. 87.

p. 95. "One black ancestor . . .," Nell Irvin Painter, *The History of White People.* New York: W. W. Norton & Co, 2010, pp. 388–99.

p. 95. From being depicted as children to being depicted as a dangerous animal, Paula Giddings, *When and Where I Enter: The Impact of Black Women on Race and Sex in America.* New York: William Morrow and Company, 1984.

p. 95. On "polygenesis," Young, *Bunk,* pp. 166, 165.

p. 97. Diversity on the other side of the species line, see pattrice jones, "Eros and the Mechanisms of Eco-Defense," in *Ecofeminism: Feminist Intersec- tions with Other Animals and the Earth.* New York: Bloomsbury, 2014, pp. 91–108.

p. 98. "A white man's country," Painter, *The History of White People,* p. 107.

p. 99. Coontz on self-reliance, *The Way We Never Were,* p. 63.

p. 99. Generous subsidies from banks, Coontz: "Every American gets 'free stuff' from government. . . . And a 2012 *New York Times* report calculated that federal and state governments had given away $170 billion in tax breaks and incentives to businesses without demanding any accountability as to whether they actually produced long-term jobs or even stayed around long enough to make up for the tax losses the communities incurred." *The Way We Never Were*, pp. xxvi–xxvii.

p. 99. Taylor quoting Michael Oliver, Sunaura Taylor, *Beast of Burden: Animal and Disability Liberation*. New York and London: The New Press, 2017, p. 107.

p. 99. "The language of dependency . . .," Taylor, *Beasts of Burden*. p. 171.

pp. 99, 101. Most of us are dependent on a huge support network . . ." paraphrase of Taylor, *Beasts of Burden*, p. 209.

p. 100. Shearing off chicken's beaks, Peter Singer, *Animal Liberation*, second edition. New York: New York Review of Books, 1990, p. 102.

p. 100. Fifty percent of pigs were lame at the time of slaughter, Temple Grandin, "The Importance of Measurement to Improve the Welfare of Livestock, Poultry, and Fish," in *Improving Animal Welfare, 2 Edition: A Practical Approach,* edited by Temple Grandin. Oxford, CAB International, 2015, p. 16.

p. 101. "Highest domestic terrorism investigation priority," *https://www. gpo.gov/fdsys/pkg/CHRG-108shrg98179/html/CHRG-108shrg98179.htm* and *https://www.fbi.gov/stats-services/publications/terrorism-2002-2005*

p. 101. Skewed priorities of the 1950s. *Color of Law,* p. 148.

p. 103. "First" sites usually refer to those that are relevant to white history, Roxanne Dunbar-Ortiz, *An Indigenous Peoples' History of the United States.* Boston: Beacon Press, 2014, p. 9.

p. 103. Manisha Sinha, *The Slave's Cause: A History of Abolition.* New Haven, CT: Yale University Press, 2016, p. 586.

p. 103. Black efforts at memory-keeping that centered on emancipation, Cecilia Elizabeth O'Leary, *To Die For: The Paradox of American Patriotism.* Princeton: Princeton University Press, 1999.

p. 103. Douglas A. Blackmon, *Slavery By Another Name: The Re-Enslavement of Black Americans from the Civil War to World War II.* New York: Anchor Books, 2008.

p. 103. Michelle Alexander, *The New Jim Crow: Mass Incarceration in the Age of Colorblindness*. New York: The New Press, 2010, 2012, pp. 11, 1.

p. 105. Faith in political progress may prevent recognizing the erosion of democratic protections. Timothy Snyder, "What Can European History Teach Us About Trump's America?" *https://www.youtube.com/watch?v=6nEmBmGK5kM*; Steven Levitsky and Daniel Ziblatt, *How Democracies Die*. New York: Crown, 2018.

p. 105. "a troubling fondness for other authoritarians," *https://www.nytimes.com/2018/01/10/opinion/trumps-how-democracies-die.html?action=click&pgtype=Homepage&clickSource=story-heading&module=opinion-c-col-left-region&region=opinion-c-col-left-region&WT.nav=opinion-c-col-left-region&_r=0*.

CHAPTER 6

p. 114. Research from Emory University and Stanford University, C. D. Cameron, B. K. Payne, "Escaping affect: how motivated emotion regulation creates insensitivity to mass suffering." *J Pers Soc Psychol* 2011; 100: 1–15.

p. 114. Simone Weil, "Reflections on the Right Use of School Studies with a View to the Love of God," in *Waiting on God*. London: Collins Books, 1951, p. 75.

p. 115. Caring was seen as "weak" politically, Coontz, *The Way We Never Were*, pp. 63, 65.

p. 116. European migrant crisis, *https://www.politico.eu/article/europe-migration-migrants-are-here-to-stay-refugee-crisis*.

p. 116. Zygmunt Bauman, *Strangers at the Door*. London: Polity Press, 2016.

p. 116. "The Trump Effect," 2016 the Southern Poverty Law Center, *https://www.splcenter.org/20160413/trump-effect-impact-presidential-campaign-our-nations-schools*.

p. 117. Brigid Brophy, "The Rights of Animals," *Sunday Times*, October 1965. Reprinted in *Don't Never Forget: Collected Views and Reviews*. New York: Holt, Rinehart and Winston, 1966.

p. 118. David Foster Wallace, "Consider the Lobster" reprinted in *Consider the Lobster and Other Essays*. New York: Little, Brown & Company, 2006, p. 246.

p. 119. Wallace on the words by which we refer to dead animals who become meat, "Consider the Lobster," footnote 15, p. 247.

p. 120. 130,000 chickens die hourly, *http://www.ansc.purdue.edu/faen/poultry%20facts.html.*

p. 120. As many as a million chickens per year dropped into boiling water alive, *http://usda.mannlib.cornell.edu/MannUsda/viewDocumentInfo.do?documentID=1497.*

p. 120. Dr. John Webster, *Animal Welfare: A Cool Eye Toward Eden*. Hoboken, NJ: Wiley-Blackwell, 1995.

p. 121. Fishes are capable of suffering, *https://www.nytimes.com/2016/05/15/opinion/fishes-have-feelings-too.html?ref=opinion&_r=3.*

p. 121. For each farmed fish more than 100 wild-caught fishes die, *http://www.countinganimals.com/the-fish-we-kill-to-feed-the-fish-we-eat.*

p. 121. Both a victim and a perpetrator, *https://www.animalsandsociety.org/human-animal-studies/society-and-animals-journal/articles-on-animal-abuse-and-human-violence/bullying-animal-abuse-connection.*

p. 123. "Who benefits when those struggling for a better world end up fighting with each other?" Lori Gruen, *http://america.aljazeera.com/opinions/2015/7/samuel-dubose-cecil-the-lion-and-the-ethics-of-avowal.html.*

p. 125. Joan Baez, "action is the antidote to despair," *https://www.rollingstone.com/music/features/joan-baez-old-folk-at-home-the-rolling-stone-interview-19830414.*

CHAPTER 7

p. 138 Mirah Curzer blog post, *https://thecoffeelicious.com/how-to-stayoutraged-without-losing-your-mind-fc0c41aa68f3.*

p. 138 Meditation and exercise reduce depression and inflammation, T. W. Pace et al., "Effect of compassion meditation on neuroendocrine, innate immune and behavioral responses to psychosocial stress." *Psychoneuroendocrinology* 2009; 34: 87–98; M. L. Kohut et al., "Aerobic exercise, but not flexibility/resistance exercise, reduces serum IL-18, CRP, and IL-6 independent of beta-blockers, BMI, and psychosocial factors in older adults." *Brain Behav Immun* 2006; 20: 201–9.

p. 139 Stress and depression linked to systemic inflammation, S. K. Lutgendorf et al., "Life stress, mood disturbance, and elevated interleukin-6 in healthy older women." *J Gerontol A Biol Sci Med Sci* 1999; 54: M434–9; J. A. Pasco et al., "Association of high-sensitivity C-reactive protein with de novo major depression." *Br J Psychiatry* 2010; 197: 372–7; D. Gimeno et al., "Associations of C-reactive protein and interleukin-6 with cognitive symptoms of depression: 12-year follow-up of the Whitehall II study." *Psychol Med* 2009; 39: 413–23.

p. 139 Inflammation as cause of depression, M. Berk et al., "So depression is an inflammatory disease, but where does the inflammation come from?" *BMC Med* 2013; 11: 200.

p. 140. Blood levels of arachidonic acid related to meat consumption, B. S. Rett, "Increasing dietary linoleic acid does not increase tissue arachidonic acid content in adults consuming Western-type diets: a systematic review." *Nutr Metab (Lond)* 2011, 8, 36; G. H. Johnson, K. Fritsche, "Effect of dietary linoleic acid on markers of inflammation in healthy persons: A systematic review of randomized controlled trials." *Journal of the Academy of Nutrition and Dietetics* 2012; 112: 1029–41.

p. 141. Oleocanthal in olive oil reduces inflammation, L. Parkinson et al., "Oleocanthal, a phenolic derived from virgin olive oil: a review of the beneficial effects on inflammatory disease." *Int J Mol Sci* 2014; 15: 12323–34.

p. 141. High blood glucose levels promote oxidative stress and inflammation, A. Ceriello et al., "Meal-induced oxidative stress and low-density lipoprotein oxidation in diabetes: the possible role of hyperglycemia." *Metabolism* 1999; 48: 1503–8.

p. 141. Fiber-rich carbohydrates may lower depression, J. E. Gangwisch et al., "High glycemic index diet as a risk factor for depression: analyses from the Women's Health Initiative." *Am J Clin Nutr* 2015.

p. 142. Quercetin can inhibit the enzyme responsible for degrading serotonin, Y. Bandaruk et al., "Cellular uptake of quercetin and luteolin and their effects on monoamine oxidase-A in human neuroblastoma SH-SY5Y cells." *Toxicol Rep* 2014; 1: 639–49.

p. 142. Eating fruits and vegetables related to happiness, B. A. White et al., "Many apples a day keep the blues away—daily experiences of negative and positive affect and food consumption in young adults. "*Br J Health Psychol* 2013; 18: 782–98.

p.142. Estrogen alleviates depression in postmenopausal women, S. Grigoriadis et al., "Role of estrogen in the treatment of depression." *Am J Ther* 2002; 9: 503–9.

p. 142. Soy isoflavones reduced depression similar to antidepressants, R. E. Estrella et al., "Effects of antidepressants and soybean association in depressive menopausal women." *Acta Pol Pharm* 2014; 71: 323–7.

P. 142. Isoflavones lower depression in women, M. Messina et al., "Evaluation of the potential antidepressant effects of soybean isoflavones." *Menopause* 2016; 23: 1348–60.

p. 143. Isoflavones equivalent to one cup of soy milk lower depression in women, A. Hirose et al., "Low-dose isoflavone aglycone alleviates psychological symptoms of menopause in Japanese women: a randomized, double-blind, placebo-controlled study." *Arch Gynecol Obstet* 2015.

p.143. Soyfoods linked to lower risk for prostate cancer, C. C. Applegate et al., "Soy Consumption and the Risk of Prostate Cancer: An Updated Systematic Review and Meta-Analysis."*Nutrients* 2018; 10.

p. 143. Low vitamin B12, vitamin D, omega-3 fats linked to depression, S. Motsinger et al., "Vitamin D intake and mental health-related quality of life in older women: the Iowa Women's Health Study." *Maturitas* 2012; 71: 267–73; K. M. Appleton et al., "Effects of n-3 long-chain polyunsaturated fatty acids on depressed mood: systematic review of published trials." *Am J Clin Nutr* 2006; 84: 1308–16; K. A. Skarupski et al., "Longitudinal association of vitamin B-6, folate, and vitamin B-12 with depressive symptoms among older adults over time." *Am J Clin Nutr* 2010; 92: 330–5.

p.144. Putting meat-eaters on vegetarian diet can improve mood, B. L. Beezhold et al., "Restriction of meat, fish, and poultry in omnivores improves mood: a pilot randomized controlled trial." *Nutr J* 2012; 11: 9.

p. 144. Air pollution associated with depression, Y. H. Lim et al., "Air pollution and symptoms of depression in elderly adults." *Environ Health Perspect* 2012; 120: 1023–8.

p. 144. Bacteria and plant-derived oils may be linked to improved mood, B. J. Park et al., "The physiological effects of Shinrin-yoku (taking in the forest atmosphere or forest bathing): evidence from field experiments in 24 forests across Japan." *Environ Health Prev Med* 2010; 15: 18–26.

p. 144. Climate change, biodiversity and mental health, "Connecting Global Priorities—Biodiversity and Human Health," World Health Organization and Secretariat of the Convention on Biological Diversity, 2015.

CHAPTER 8

p. 160. Protein protects bone health, R. G. Munger et al., "Prospective study of dietary protein intake and risk of hip fracture in postmenopausal women." *Am J Clin Nutr* 1999; 69: 147–52; D. L. Thorpe et al., "Effects of meat consumption and vegetarian diet on risk of wrist fracture over 25 years in a cohort of peri- and postmenopausal women." *Public Health Nutr* 2008; 11: 564–72; J. H. Promislow et al., "Protein consumption and bone mineral density in the elderly: the Rancho Bernardo Study." *Am J Epidemiol* 2002; 155: 636–44; A. Devine et al., "Protein consumption is an important predictor of lower limb bone mass in elderly women." *Am J Clin Nutr* 2005; 81: 1423–8.

p. 160. Research supports quality of plant protein, V. R. Young, P. L. Pellett, "Plant proteins in relation to human protein and amino acid nutrition." *Am J Clin Nutr* 1994; 59: 1203S–1212S.

p. 161. 10-year anniversary edition, Frances Moore Lappé. *Diet for a Small Planet.* New York: Ballantine, 1981.

p. 162. Fruits and vegetables protect bone health, S. A. New, "Intake of fruit and vegetables: implications for bone health." *Proc Nutr Soc* 2003; 62: 889–99.

ACKNOWLEDGMENTS

From the moment we started working on this book, it was embraced by an incredible team of advocates. Our agents, Stephanie Tade and Colleen Martell of the Stephanie Tade Agency, provided recommendations that helped the book take its present shape and helped us create a more effective tool for the resistance. We are grateful for their support, enthusiasm, and friendship and for their believing in this book right from the start. We have been truly amazed by and thankful for the enthusiasm we experienced in every single encounter with our publishing team. Thank you to our editors Peter Turner and Christine LeBlond at Conari/Red Wheel for their guidance, support, and unwavering commitment to producing the best book possible. A huge shout out to designer Kathryn Sky-Peck for capturing the spirit of our book so perfectly and for bringing that same spirit to the book design. Bonni Hamilton and Eryn Eaton worked with us with unwavering zeal to help us bring our book's message out into the world.

Thank you to Matt Ball, Lawrence Carter-Long, Karen Davis, Kathryn Gillespie, pattrice jones, Jo-Anne McArthur, Mia McDonald, Dawn Moncrief, lauren Ornelas, Will Potter, and Brenda Sanders for taking the time to talk with us about the issues in this book and for sharing their experiences and expertise.

Carol wants to thank her sisters Nancy and Jane who have kept her email inbox filled with all-too-relevant news articles and analyses. Nancy originated the idea of the Resistance Dinner, offering creative thoughts on draining the swamp, trumped up this and that, and all in all, helping us think about politically playing with our food. Bryanna Clark Grogan accepted the challenge of creating many of the dishes found in the Resistance Feast. We are indebted to her creativity and have benefited from it over the years as we have cooked from her recipes. We are constantly inspired by the work of so many talented vegan cooks and are grateful to Gena Hamshaw, Fran Costigan, and Allison Samson Rivers for contributing recipes to our book.

During a Facebook discussion of "dog whistles," Susan Schweik pointed out how the term implicitly animalized those being targeted.

In writing the book, Carol drew on some of her recent writings including "The Sexual Politics of Meat in the Trump Era," forthcoming from University of Nevada Press in an edited volume by Laura Wright. She thanks Laura Wright for working with her on that essay. Chapter 4 also draws on material developed for short essays featured by *Truthdig*, *Tikkun*, and *Open Democracy*. Finally, working on a new preface for the Bloomsbury Revelations edition of her 1994 book *Neither Man nor Beast* helped consolidate Carol's ideas about "Take Out Misogyny."

Carol tried out some of the ideas found in chapter 5 at the State University of New York at Fredonia in September 2017 celebrating the 100th anniversary of women's suffrage in New York State. Emily van Dette organized that convocation talk and suggested tying in her analysis of social activism of the 19th century to more recent activism. In a presentation at Animal Place's 2017 Food Justice for All conference, Carol was able to explore some of the ideas in the book and receive helpful feedback.

As always, Jane Nearing has been indefatigable in her role as a reference librarian at the Richardson (Texas) Public Library. And during a challenging deadline for the book, the wonderful women at Punk Rawk Labs sent some of their delicious cheese. Bruce Buchanan provided just the right kinds of support at just the right times. Thanks for all these kinds of nurturance!

Ginny is grateful for her community of vegan health professionals who work to promote an ethic of animal rights with compassion and scientific integrity. Thank you especially to Jack Norris, RD; Reed Mangels, PhD, RD; Anya Todd, MS, RD; Taylor Wolfram, MS, RD; Matt Ruscigno, MPH, RD; Carolyn Tampe, MS, RD; David Weinman, RD; Ed

Coffin, RD. She is indebted to the members of Berkshire Voters for Animals for including her in their advocacy for all animals through legislation. As always, she is blessed to be married to Mark Messina, best nutrition advisor, best cat dad, and best husband.

Finally, we thank you, our readers, for caring about social justice and for including this book as part of your resistance library. Together, we can make change happen. The Republic is a Dream. Nothing happens unless first a dream.

INDEX

ABOUT THE AUTHORS

Carol J. Adams is the author of the pioneering *The Sexual Politics of Meat*, which the *New York Times* called a "vegan bible," and is now in a 25th-anniversary edition. The book was named one of *Ms.* readers' 100 Best Non-Fiction Books of All Time. Carol has also written pieces for sources as diverse as the *New York Times*, the *Washington Post*, *Ms.* magazine, and *Christian Century.* She is a popular speaker on college campuses and keynoter at international conferences. She lives in Dallas with her partner and two rescued dogs. Visit Carol at *caroljadams.com*

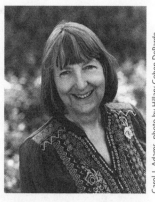

Carol J. Adams, photo by Hillary Cohen DeParde

Virginia Messina is a registered dietitian with a master's degree in public health nutrition from the University of Michigan. She is a longtime vegan who writes about vegetarian and vegan diets for the public and health professionals. She is the author of *Vegan for Her* and the coauthor of *Vegan for Life*, and her articles have appeared in a variety of popular publications including *Family Circle* magazine, *Self* magazine, and the *Encyclopedia Britannica*. Ginny lives with her husband and a group of rescued cats in Pittsfield, MA. Visit her at *TheVeganRD.com*

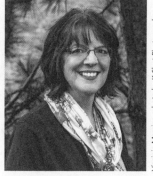

Virginia Messina, photo by K Shot Photography

TO OUR READERS